SpringerBriefs in Public Health

T0236364

For further volumes:
http://www.springer.com/series/10138

John G. Bruhn

Culture and Health Disparities

Evaluation of Interventions and Outcomes in the U.S.-Mexico Border Region

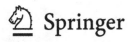
Springer

John G. Bruhn
Northern Arizona University
Flagstaff, AZ
USA

ISSN 2192-3698   ISSN 2192-3701   (electronic)
ISBN 978-3-319-06461-1   ISBN 978-3-319-06462-8   (eBook)
DOI 10.1007/978-3-319-06462-8
Springer Cham Heidelberg New York Dordrecht London

Library of Congress Control Number: 2014939407

Springer is part of Springer Science+Business Media (www.springer.com)

Of all the forms of inequality, injustice in healthcare is the most shocking and inhumane.

Dr. Martin Luther King, Jr.

Acknowledgments

Jeff Brandon, former Dean of the College of Health and Social Services at New Mexico State University, led a conference titled "Making Connections: An Interdisciplinary Conference to Address Disparities in Health Status in the American Southwest" in October, 2003 in Las Cruces, New Mexico. The purpose of the conference was to utilize the Healthy Gente/Border 2010 objectives as a framework to build a partnership between academic institutions, public agencies, practitioners, and consumers in order to reduce disparities in the Southwest Border Region.

Funding support for this conference was shared by the National Cancer Institute, Office of Women's Health (NIH), Paso de Norte Health Foundation, the New Mexico Outreach Office of the U.S.-Mexico Border Health Commission, and the New Mexico Border Health Education Training Center. Proceedings are available on CD.

Conferees identified several key principles that are necessary in order to reduce/ eliminate Border Health Disparities. These principles are: respect, trust, honesty, inclusion, reciprocation, sustainability, and capacity building. While no formal follow-up has been conducted over the decade since the conference, major challenges remain due in large part to competing problems surrounding immigration policy, border security, violence, and illegal drug abuse. Hopefully, this volume will encourage health professionals and health-care policy makers to continue to make positive gains despite the prevalence of overreaching problems.

I am indebted to Tracy Grindle for her fine skills as an editor and typist. Vince Colburn is responsible for the excellent graphic art work.

Contents

Contents

Chapter 1
The Border Region: Its Culture and Health Disparities

1.1 Introduction

Boundary lines of any type are not found in the real world itself, only in the imagination of mapmakers (Wilber 1981). There are no natural boundaries between opposites, rather boundaries are products of the way we map and edit reality.[1] We name, classify, and note differences between people, things, and events and draw dividing lines which recognize them as separate groups.[2] We can refine our perceptions further to find deeper differences, which may result in stereotypes. Stereotypes often become accepted as reality and influence our behavior toward people, things, and events that we perceive as different from our own beliefs or values. Boundaries can become barriers or obstacles when based primarily on differences between groups; but groups may also share common values, what social psychologist Muzafer Sherif termed "superordinate goals" (Sherif et al. 1961). A superordinate goal is one where people who are normally competitors or antagonists unite for mutual survival. For example, optimal health could be a superordinate goal for the U.S.-Mexico border region. Despite challenging differences in communication styles and resources the optimization of health could be an achievable goal for the border region (Murphy 1998).

---

[1] See Dear (2013), who states that without the presence of an international boundary, each pair of borderland twin cities would be instantly recognizable as a single, integrated metropolis. He shows how to think about the possibility of a border region without walls.

[2] On October 26, 2006 President George W. Bush signed H.R. 6061 into law, known as the Secure Fence Act. There is a down payment of $1.2 billion to the Department of Homeland Security marked for border security but not specifically for a border fence. As of 2010 the fence project had been completed from San Diego to Yuma. Controversy led Congress to revisit the fence plan. On March 16, 2010, President Obama stated the money would be used to upgrade current border technology. The border fence is not one continuous structure rather it is a grouping of short physical walls that stop and start, secured in between with a "virtual fence" which includes a system of sensors and cameras monitored by Border Patrol Agents. See The Border Fence (http://www.pbs.org/now/shows/432).

J. G. Bruhn, *Culture and Health Disparities*, SpringerBriefs in Public Health, DOI: 10.1007/978-3-319-06462-8_1, © The Author(s) 2014

A positive example of progress toward a superordinate goal is the development of the 10 year 2012 Border Program in the Pacific Southwest Region 9 of the Environmental Protection Agency, to protect the environment and public health of the U.S.-Mexico border region. This program was developed using the principles of sustainable development. It takes a regional approach with local input to best address environmental issues in the border region. A variety of stakeholders prioritize sustainable actions that consider the environmental needs of different border communities. As a result, successful projects include engine idle reduction activities, energy audits of manufacturing plants, a project to promote the processing of waste grease from restaurants to generate biodiesel fuel, and engine retrofits for school buses (U.S. EPA 2012).

1.1.1 U.S.-Mexico Relations

The U.S. and Mexico have a long history of cooperation on environmental and national resource issues in the border area. There are serious environmental problems but cooperative activities take place under a number of arrangements. Presidents Obama and Calderon created an Executive Steering Committee for 21st century Border Management in 2010 to spur advancements in creating a modern, secure and efficient border.

The Merida Initiative is a partnership between the U.S. and Mexico to fight organized crime and associated violence while furthering respect for human rights and the rule of law. The U.S. Congress has appropriated $1.9 billion for the Merida Initiative since it was signed into law in 2008. The scope of U.S.-Mexican relations is broad and goes beyond diplomatic and official contacts. It entails extensive commercial, cultural and educational ties. One million American citizens live in Mexico and roughly ten million Americans visit Mexico each year. More than 18,000 companies with U.S. investments have operations in Mexico, and U.S. companies have invested $145 billion in Mexico since 2000. Mexican investments in the U.S. have grown by over 35 % in the last 5 years (U.S. Dept. of State 2012; National Immigration Forum 2012).

The first program specifically targeting residents of the U.S.-Mexico border region began in the early 1940s when thousands of Mexican nationals were hired as temporary agricultural laborers to meet U.S. labor shortages during World War II. However, federal and state departments of health did not begin to focus on border health until the 1990s (U.S.-Mexico Border Health Commission 2010a, b). Early interventions focused on the surveillance and prevention of communicable diseases. In 1983 the U.S. and Mexican governments signed the La Paz Agreement on Cooperation for the Prevention and Improvement of the Environment in the Border Area and accepted a definition of the shared "border region" as the geographical area defined by 100 km (62 miles) north and south of the U.S.-Mexico border. Public Law 103-400 (1994) authorized the President of the U.S. to establish an agreement with Mexico to create a binational commission to address serious health problems in the border region.

1.2 Boundaries: The Guardians of Culture

Boundaries have several dimensions, political, geographical, physical, social, and psychological. How we perceive, interpret and respond to boundaries is influenced by our culture. Boundaries keep people together and separate others, temporarily or permanently. Boundaries determine our social networks, relationships and cross-cultural ties. Environmental factors also play a determining role in shaping the lives of distinct populations. For example, rural people differ from urban people and inner-city residents differ from suburbanites. Similarly, border residents differ from people who live in heartland regions. Martinez (1994) studied people who lived in the U.S.-Mexico borderlands analyzing how they were influenced by forces generated by the U.S.-Mexico boundary itself. He found three major cultural groups in the borderlands, Mexicans, Mexican-Americans, and Anglo Americans resulting in an array of cross-boundary relationships and lifestyles. Martinez explained that the borderlands culture is a product of forces and influences generated by the boundary itself, by regional phenomenon from each nation, and by the transculturation shared by Mexicans and Americans. Pastor and Castaneda (1988) found that the meaning and usefulness of boundaries can vary situationally from an abstraction and inconvenience to one of control and segregation. When the U.S.-Mexico border region is viewed and treated as a political boundary, issues of control and segregation have created disagreements between the two nations. Nonetheless, U.S. and Mexican communities on both sides of the border have collaborated on joint health improvement activities for many decades.

The purpose here is to better understand the influence the U.S.-Mexico boundary has on the lives of borderlanders especially on their health and well-being. Specifically the objective of this text is to identify effective and promising culturally appropriate public health interventions that will address the continuing health issues of communities along the U.S.-Mexico border and maintain progress toward the optimization of health for the region.

1.3 Border Culture[3]

The U.S.-Mexico border region is one of sharp socioeconomic contrasts, continuous social change and rapid economic and population growth. The border extends in length for about 2,000 miles from the Pacific Ocean to the Gulf of Mexico. This 130 mile wide strip may be North America's fastest growing region (see

---

[3] Culture has been defined in many ways. We use the well-known anthropological consensus definition: "culture consists of patterned ways of thinking, feeling, and reacting, acquired and transmitted by symbols, constituting the distinctive achievements of human groups...." (Kluckhohn 1951).

Fig. 1.1 The U.S.-Mexico border. *Source* Border Health: Challenges for the United States and Mexico. Edited by J. G. Bruhn and J. E. Brandon. Garland Publishing, Inc. New York, 1997

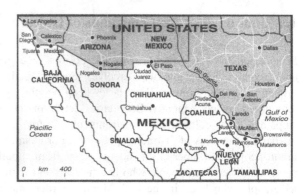

Fig. 1.1). The border region is home to more than 12 million people—by 2020 the population along the border is expected to double to more than 24 million people (EPA 2011). In 2008 there were 11.4 million Mexican immigrants to the U.S., about half of whom were unauthorized; many settle in traditional destination states like Texas and California and in the 14 pairs of sister cities divided by the border (Terrazas 2010). The U.S.-Mexico border does not separate distinct cultures from one another. It is an interactive border. Cities often have more in common with their sister cities across the border than with cities on their own side of the border (Bruhn 1997). The communities along the border are economically and socially interdependent with some one million legal north bound crossings daily in 2008 (Rodriquez-Saldana 2005; Homedes and Ugalde 2003). Valenzuela (1992) describes the border as a "floating population" indicating its mobility and interdependence.

Seeking a better life and economic opportunities encourage hundreds of thousands of job seekers from Mexico to migrate every year to live in tarpaper and cinderblock slums near factory gates. They are willing to work long hours for low pay—from $5 to $7 a day with few, if any, benefits. U.S. companies have set up assembly plants,—maquiladoras—on the Mexican side to tap this pool of cheap labor. About 2,500 maquiladoras have been key to U.S. global competiveness (Smith and Malkin 1997; Gerber 2009; DOT 2012).[4]

The border economy is flourishing due to the North American Free Trade Agreement (NAFTA) signed in 1993 whereby the economies of the U.S., Canada, and Mexico would become increasingly integrated. A more open economy and low wages have made this region attractive to global investors throughout the world (Smith and Malkin 1997).

---

[4] See Good Neighbor Environmental Board (GNEB) and Environmental Advisors Across Borders (2010). National Service Center for Environmental Publications, Pub. No. EPA 130-R-10-001,nscep@bps-lmt.com . The GNEB is an independent U.S. Presidential advisory committee that meets twice yearly in various U.S. border communities and also in Washington D.C. to inform the President and Congress about environmental issues along the U.S.-Mexico border.

Paradoxically the U.S.-Mexico border region is one of the poorest in the U.S. Ganster and Lorey (2008) point out that "if the border region were the 51st state" it would rank:

- Last in access to health care
- Second in death due to hepatitis
- Third in deaths related to diabetes mellitus
- Last in per capita income
- First in the number of school children living in poverty
- First in the number of children who do not have health insurance (pp. 172–174)

1.3.1 Social and Kin Networks

Informal networks provide mechanisms that border residents use to cope with the stresses of rapid population growth, low income, and health risks. During times of stress cross-border networks become viable links to social, economic and psychological survival. People seek goods and services on whichever side of the border offers the best value and most culturally comfortable service (Ingram et al. 1995). The ability of people to maintain ties, bridge differences, forge informal networks, and develop a common culture underlies the growth and economic success of the border region.

The U.S. border states with their Mexican culture, Spanish language, Latino institutions, and economic ties to Mexico create a context that promotes transnational lives. Mexicans along the border use the resources and skills they bring from Mexico to address issues in U.S. communities and family life. Even as they are acculturated to U.S. society, the families maintain ties to Mexico and as they rear children, go to school, vote, and participate in communities in the U.S. Instead of loosening their connection or trading one identity for another, Mexicans who live in the U.S. borderlands forge social relationships, earn livelihoods, and exercise their rights across borders (Marquez and Romo 2008).

The kin network that links binational families facilitates cross-border exchange. Firefighters, police, and disaster resource operations regularly cross the border for emergencies. Public health officials have developed lines of communication to exchange equipment, diagnoses, and sometimes patients. Academic and government researchers exchange information and peer review comments (Ingram et al. 1995). The border area is also grounded in a Mexican culture of strong family values, historical legacies, and the blending of English and Spanish languages (Marquez and Romo 2008).

The borderlands reflect the incorporation of resident Mexicans as well as a continuous process of back and forth migration. Jobs on both sides promote binational commerce and social gatherings involving family members from both countries. Culture and kinship relations help Mexican-origin residents in the U.S. lessen the impact of racial and socioeconomic discrimination and foster opportunities for recognition and incorporation (Bastida 2001). Kinship networks help to link individuals who seek social mobility in the U.S. to stable social structures on both sides of the border. Milardo (1988) writes:

> Families live in an elaborate system of interaction where they create ties of varying complexity and strength with an array of other individuals, other families, and larger social complexities. Families are profoundly influenced by this web of ties and they are active agents in modifying and adapting these communities of personal relationships to meet ever-changing circumstances (pp. 13–14).

Bastida (2001) found that kinship networks were essential for lowering and possibly eliminating the high risk behaviors associated with undocumented immigration and finding work. Kinship networks protect migrants from becoming visible to authorities and apprehended. Kin networks help offer protection against unscrupulous border traffickers and other exploitative relationships. A number of immigrant women who succeeded in their migration depended on embedded kinship networks for their survival, stability, and long-term adjustment (Bastida 2001).

1.4 Border Health

There is a dark side to border culture as well. The transitory nature of border lifestyle and the protection of anonymity has enabled illegal activity associated with drugs and immigration in particular, to predominate daily life. The attention of border dwellers has become focused on personal safety which is a diversion from the prevention and treatment of physical, mental, and environmental health problems. The region has a limited health infrastructure. Nonetheless there is cross-border utilization of health care services in Mexico by U.S. residents living near the border and Mexican immigrants, including the undocumented, who use health services in the U.S. (Chavez et al. 1985; Byrd and Law 2009). Border residents have disproportionally high levels of obesity, diabetes mellitus, cervical cancer and communicable diseases such as tuberculosis. Hispanics living on the border are the poorest and have limited access to health care and, in general, have a lower quality of health compared to non-Hispanics (U.S.-Mexico Border Health Commission 2010a, b).

According to the U.S. Environmental Protection Agency, poorly planned industrial and population growth in the region has resulted in high levels of air pollution, water scarcity, water-and-land contamination, inadequate solid waste and sewage systems, and degradation of natural resources and ecosystems (Homedes and Ugalde 2009).

Border residents have high levels of poverty, low education levels, and high rates of uninsured individuals, compared to national averages. Most border hospitals report high levels of uncompensated care. In some hospitals as much as two thirds of total operating costs are for uncompensated care for illegal immigrants (Ruark and Martin 2009). The majority of the uninsured reside in border counties where the percent uninsured ranges between 25 and 38 % (Homedes and Ugalde 2009).

Table 1.1 shows the recent ten leading causes of death for U.S. and Mexican border states.

The U.S. and Mexico have the first two causes of death in common, that is, diseases of the heart and malignant neoplasms. Diabetes mellitus, liver disease and cirrhosis, and influenza and pneumonia are also among the top ten shared causes for mortality. The U.S. border states have more deaths from Alzheimer's disease, unintentional injuries, and suicide than the Mexican border states, while the Mexican border states have more deaths from homicide and perinatal conditions than the U.S. border states (PAHO 2012).

1.5 Health Disparities and Culture

Health disparities are not new nor are they unique to Mexico, the United States, or their borders (Williams 2011). There has been evidence internationally for several centuries of a link between nonmedical factors and health and health care outcomes (Gibbons 2005). *Health disparities can be defined as inequalities that exist when members of certain population groups do not benefit from the same health status as other groups.* (See entire issue of *Health Affairs* 27(2)2008).[5] A legal definition is "a population is a health disparity population if there is a significant disparity in the overall rate of disease incidence, prevalence, morbidity, mortality or survival rates in the population as compared to the health status of the general population" (Minority Health and Health Disparities Research and Education Act of 2000).

Defining and measuring a disparity is a prerequisite for resolving or ameliorating it.[6] While definitions of disparities are not standardized and multiple definitions are in current use, disparities are generally considered to be population differences in (1) environmental exposures, (2) health care access, utilization, or quality, (3) health status (longevity),[7] or (4) health outcomes (Carter-Pokras and Baquet 2002).

---

[5] For additional perspectives on disparities see Schnittker and McLeod (2005). Also, Braveman (2006). Also, Bleich et al. (2012)

[6] The terms "health disparities" and "health inequalities" will be used interchangeably here.

[7] See Bergner and Rothman (1987). Health status is not commonly understood because the term "health status" has not been clearly defined and a consensus agreed to. Few have operationalized the term so that it can be used to access the level of health among a group of people. Length of life is the ultimate measure of health status where acute illnesses that are potentially fatal is concerned. In chronic illnesses where palliative therapies may prevent further deterioration the relevant measure of health status will include aspects of health other than the length of life.

Table 1.1 Ten leading causes of death, United States and Mexican border states, 2007 and 2008

U.S. border states (2007)		Mexican border states (2008)	
Cause of death	Mortality per 100,000 population	Cause of death	Mortality per 100,000 population
1. Diseases of the heart	162.5–168.8	1. Diseases of the heart	78.0–112.2
2. Malignant neoplasms	150.5–164.4	2. Malignant neoplasm	52.9–76.5
3. Unintentional injuries	31.8–67.5	3. Diabetes mellitus	45.0–87.4
4. Cerebrovascular diseases	34.8–41.0	4. Homicides	7.6–75.2
5. Chronic lower respiratory diseases	33.9–44.9	5. Unintentional injuries	25.9–55.0
6. Diabetes mellitus	18.3–34.2	6. Cerebrovascular diseases	20.4–29.7
7. Alzheimer's disease	16.3–32.4	7. Chronic liver disease and cirrhosis	17.6–29.8
8. Influenza and pneumonia	13.5–17.9	8. Influenza and pneumonia	8.2–15.8
9. Chronic liver disease and cirrhosis	10.6–18.9	9. Conditions originating in the perinatal period	7.4–16.3
10. Suicide	9.9–20.4	10. Chronic obstructive pulmonary diseases	9.1–16.5

Sources United States, Centers for Disease Control and Prevention. Deaths, percent of total deaths, and death rates for the 15 leading causes of death: United States and each state (Internet); 2007. Available at http://www.cdc.gov/nchs/data/dvs/LCWK9_2007.pdf. Accessed on 29 December 2011. Mexico, Sistema Nacional de Informacion en Salud. Principales causas de mortalidad general por entidad federativa (Internet); 2008. Available at: http://sinais.salud.gob. mx/mortalidad. Accessed on 29 December 2011. Reproduced from *Health in the Americas*, FAHO, 2012, p. 707

1.5.1 Causes of Disparities

The root "causes" of health disparities are numerous and relate to individual behaviors, provider knowledge and attitudes, organization of the health care system and social and cultural values (Thomas et al. 2004). In particular racial and ethnic minorities in the U.S. have been burdened with deep and persistent history-based health disparities (Byrd and Clayton 2003). These disparities reflect socioeconomic differences, inadequate access to quality health care and direct or indirect discrimination (Byrd and Clayton 2003). In addition, there is evidence that cultural norms regarding diet and exercise, for example, contribute to lifestyles and behaviors associated with risk factors for chronic disease. Therefore, efforts toward the reduction of health disparities must address the intersection of social, cultural and environmental factors beyond the simple cause-effect model (Thomas et al. 2004). Achieving greater equity may do more for health than perfecting the technology of care (Woolf et al. 2004). Furthermore, interventions that address "deep culture" (e.g. beliefs, values, and habits) as opposed to "surface culture" (e.g. language, food, music) are more effective in addressing the multiple level determinants of health that underlie disparities (Resnicow and Braithwaite 2001).

Adler and Newman (2002) indicate that the most fundamental causes of health disparities are socioeconomic, traditionally defined by education, income, and occupation (also Wilkinson 1996). These are powerful determinants of health that are not likely to have a direct causal effect but serve as proxies for other determinants. It is not feasible to isolate socioeconomic factors that contribute to health disparities because social systems are active, ongoing and complexly interactive. The investigative model used, therefore, must be broad enough to collect data from a variety of perspectives using various methods that yield information about a moving social system. Because of the economic limitations to carrying out such an endeavor, it must be collaborative and framed by long-term realistic goals for the border region (Bilheimer and Sisk 2008). Indeed, the nature of disparities will change with the changing lifecycle of the municipos and the region as a whole.

1.5.2 The Effect of Aging on Border Disparities

Peach (2012) has carefully outlined the effects of the current and continuing aging of the border states, counties and municipios. The aging of the border population is a reflection of national trends in Mexico and the U.S. Aging will affect future population growth, the size and growth of the labor force, the distribution of income and wealth, the consumption of goods, the demand for housing, and the volume of imports and exports.

Age also influences the demand for public services, particularly education and health care and environmental issues will become more complex. National policy responses to key issues such as trade, energy, immigration, health care and education will also reshape the border region. Changes in the economy will have different effects on different economic groups. The border counties and municipios are not homogeneous and have different age distributions. Aging will change the political environment nationally and in the borderlands. Aging will, in short, call for a reassessment of policies and strategies to close the gap in existing disparities and prevent new disparities from developing.

1.6 Eliminating/Reducing Health Disparities

Eliminating health disparities by preventing them is a fundamental, though not always explicit, goal of public health research and practice (Adler and Rehkopf 2008). Definitions of disparities suggest that a group's health status can be compared to the majority of a population, the population average, or the healthiest group. Most research has focused on disparities due to race and ethnicity or disparities due to socioeconomic resources. Differences in biological potential have been raised in relation to racial and ethnic health disparities, suggesting that these are differences rather than disparities. Health disparities can result from both biological differences and social differences (Adler and Rehkopf 2008).

An important factor in serving Mexican patients is their understanding of, and the definitions of, health and illness. Mexicans do not define health as a condition, but as complex interactions between personal beliefs, cultural values, and physical, emotional, and spiritual factors. Mexicans in the border region seek health services in a number of different ways depending on their level of acculturation, education, financial resources, and the particular illness or condition at hand. Kinship is an important concept with respect to reducing health disparities in health care among Mexicans. They commonly seek assistance from "primary helpers" (family members, friends, neighbors, curanderos, or other healers). The Hispanic concept of health tends to emphasize psychosomatic attributes of illness as a reflection of body/mind equilibrium, characterized by physical, mental and spiritual balance. Mexicans commonly depend more on their family for health care advice and emotional support and less on health care professionals (Ruiz-Beltran and Kamau 2001). Disparities related to the access and utilization of health services that can be observed in the border region are substantial. Sometimes disparities exist within a family or between family members. Generational status, educational status, language skills and strength of kinship ties are key to understanding the underutilization of health services.

Differences can widen and deepen to become inequalities (Herbert et al. 2008). For example, the loss of a job for a person who is an ethnic minority or blue collar worker may greatly affect the health services available to him when unemployed—a difference can become a disparity. We need persuasive data on the causes of disparities to construct pathways or mechanisms for interventions to alleviate their occurrence (Kumanyika 2012). Pathways are not always direct, linear, or uniform, therefore, eliminating disparities completely is not realistic. It seems more realistic to establish a goal of reducing or preventing disparities

Table 1.2 Focus areas and expected outcomes for healthy border 2010 agenda

Access to care: Reduce the population lacking access to a primary health provider

Cancer: Reduce breast cancer and cervical cancer mortality

Diabetes mellitus: Reduce both the mortality rate of diabetes and the need for hospitalization

Environmental health: Improve household access to sewage disposal and reduce hospital admissions for acute pesticide poisoning

HIV/AIDS: Reduce the number of cases

Immunization and infectious diseases: Expand immunization coverage for young children; reduce the incidence of hepatitis and tuberculosis

Injury prevention: Reduce mortality from motor vehicle crashes and childhood mortality from injuries

Maternal, Infant, and Child Health: Reduce overall infant mortality and infant deaths due to congenital defects, improve prenatal care, and reduce teenage pregnancy rates

Mental Health: Reduce suicide mortality

Oral Health: Improve access to oral health care

Respiratory Diseases: Reduce the rate of hospitalization for asthma

Source Border lives: Health status in the U.S.-Mexico Border Region, U.S.-Mexico Border Health Commission (2010, pp. 13–14)

rather than eliminating them. Many of the root causes of disparities are embedded in the deep culture of societies and groups. Intervention and culture changes would have to address the history of distrust, values, and create new meaningful, effective paths of health communication (Freimuth and Quinn 2004).

The U.S.-Mexico Border Health Commission developed an agenda for 2010 and projected it to 2020 to address deep culture disparities that transcend the ten causes of death previously presented in Table 1.1.

Table 1.2 shows the focus areas and expected outcomes for the Commission's Healthy Border Agenda for 2010. These areas are limited to a small number of variables for which data are currently available or are expected to be available in the near future. Of note are disparities in oral health and mental health which are often neglected in disparity interventions.

1.7 A Social System Roadmap for Preventing and Reducing Health Disparities

The social and health needs and disparities along the U.S.-Mexico border continue to grow in complexity and severity despite numerous binational conferences, commissions, and agreements (U.S.-Mexico Border Health Commission 2003, 2010a, b). Despite advocacy and information-sharing efforts, effective and sustained mechanisms for consensus-building on how best to intervene in various health problems, share "best practices," and replicate effective interventions, have not been widely developed and used. The understanding and resolution of the political, cultural, and social impediments to many common health issues remain substantial on both sides of the border. (Homedes and Ugalde 2003, 2009; Ganster and Lorey 2008). Too much emphasis continues to be placed on "downstream" problems such as morbidity and mortality rates, the use and non-use of health services, and disease intervention with a curative focus (Campbell 1974; Gehlert et al. 2008). Kozel et al. (2006) propose a transformational process for redirecting the border health agenda "upstream," that is, one that centers around primary prevention and risk factor reduction and uses political and economic interventions such as the increased taxation of tobacco, lobbying, and increased media involvement, and public education to create and sustain broader health behavior change.

There is a need for rigorous research that is designed to evaluate the effectiveness of public health interventions (Glasgow et al. 1999, 2004). Although there is a large body of evidence that demonstrates the efficacy of behavioral interventions, the translation of research findings into practice is limited by the lack of useful models, incomplete methods, and the type and quality of data available (Glasgow et al. 2004). Much of what we have learned about the effectiveness of health interventions is limited by traditional disciplinary models and methods such as the linear cause-effect approach, while understanding the nature of the border and interventions to ameliorate its health and social problems requires a systems or ecological approach. What we need to know about the border, its problems, and program successes and failures is restricted by the kinds of questions we ask and the kinds of data we gather to answer them (Bruhn and Rebach 2007; Bruhn 2009; Bastida et al. 2008; Diez Roux 2012; Rashid et al. 2009; Braveman et al. 2011).

Glanz and Bishop (2010) point out that interventions to reduce health disparities require behavior change at multiple levels. It is their opinion that public health and health promotion interventions are most likely to be effective if they are framed with an ecological perspective. Interventions should not only be targeted at individuals but also interpersonal, organizational and environmental factors influencing health behavior. Dakubo (2010) explains, "with growing criticism of the individualistic focus of the biomedical model of health and its failure to respond to the complex and structural determinants of poor health, a "new" public health emerged in the mid-1970s. The focus of this new public health was to shift the focus from the individual to a multi-causal, socio-ecological approach to health, taking into account the interaction of social, environmental, psychosocial and other factors in producing ill health" (p. 21). The ecological perspective makes use of systems thinking, it recognizes that health disparities are nested at various levels (interpersonal, organizational, community, and public policy), and cannot be changed through uni-dimensional interventions (McLeroy et al. 1988).

The ecological model considers multiple levels of influence and emphasizes environmental and policy contexts of behavior while incorporating social and psychological influences (Sellis et al. 2008). There are four core principles of the ecological perspective: (1) multiple levels of factors influence health behaviors; (2) influences interact across levels; (3) multi-level interventions should be the most effective in changing behavior; and (4) the ecological model is most effective when it is behavior-specific such as tobacco control or diabetes self-management (Sellis et al. 2008).

Diez Roux (2011) notes that the causes of health disparities requires understanding how the dynamic relationships between factors at different levels of organization results in the emergence of health differences across groups. The key question is understanding how dynamic relationships among factors generate the disparities that we see. Link and Phelan (1995) note that, if risk factors are not more broadly contextualized we run the risk of imposing individually-based intervention strategies that are ineffective and miss opportunities to adopt broad-based interventions that could produce reductions in health disparities.

1.8 Issues in Assessing the Effectiveness of Border Health Interventions

Data on health problems along the U.S.-Mexico border come primarily from 80 municipios in six Mexican states and 48 counties in four U.S. states. These data often lack common definitions and common data elements, may be gathered under different surveillance timelines and with different frequencies, and therefore have limited usefulness in planning and implementing interventions. The lack of data rigor can impede generalizability and distort important differences due to demography, culture, and/or disparities. For example, it is not possible to directly compare death rates in the U.S. and Mexico without considering that the majority population of Mexico is younger than the U.S. Similarly, the U.S. border region has lower rates of communicable diseases and some chronic diseases compared to the adjacent border region of Mexico, despite sharing some common risk factors. Without greater cross-border refinement of data content and coordination it will be difficult to identify and intervene in reducing risks and disparities. Available data and its current forms often determines what we study rather than build a data system focused on measurable variables that will yield data to fill existing knowledge gaps, and present new questions.

Available data not only influences what we research and evaluate but data are a product of the disciplinary perspective of the persons who gather it. Researchers in medicine and public health have grown used to thinking about determinants of individual health, or more broadly about the health of populations, that they have neglected intermediate forms of social organization, such as communities and groups, especially the interaction between these levels (see Table 1.3). Different levels of analysis produce different data about health between the individual and population determinants as well as between different groups within a given population.

In recent literature public health researchers have reconsidered the contribution of social epidemiology. Many large scale studies have fallen short of expectations in identifying specific risk factors for disease onset and recurrence and many interventions to change individual high risk behaviors for certain diseases have been only minimally successful. Glass (2000) believes that these limitations are due to risk factors being viewed as discrete, voluntary, and individually modifiable lifestyle choices, detached from the social context in which behaviors arise. Syme (2004) stated that successes in smoking cessation have come about when they have been designed and implemented using a multipronged, multilevel, multidisciplinary approach. These approaches involve not only information but also

Table 1.3 Algorithm for studying behavior at the individual, group, and population levels of analysis

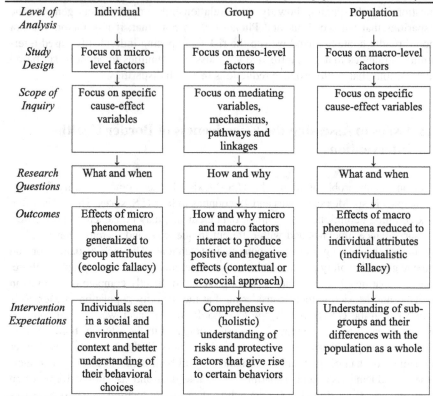

Level of Analysis	Individual	Group	Population
Study Design	Focus on micro-level factors	Focus on meso-level factors	Focus on macro-level factors
Scope of Inquiry	Focus on specific cause-effect variables	Focus on mediating variables, mechanisms, pathways and linkages	Focus on specific cause-effect variables
Research Questions	What and when	How and why	What and when
Outcomes	Effects of micro phenomena generalized to group attributes (ecologic fallacy)	How and why micro and macro factors interact to produce positive and negative effects (contextual or ecosocial approach)	Effects of macro phenomena reduced to individual attributes (individualistic fallacy)
Intervention Expectations	Individuals seen in a social and environmental context and better understanding of their behavioral choices	Comprehensive (holistic) understanding of risks and protective factors that give rise to certain behaviors	Understanding of sub-groups and their differences with the population as a whole

Source Bruhn (2009, p. 9)

regulations and laws, mass media programs, workplace rules, and better environmental engineering and design. Inevitably, he said, "We in public health need to think across disciplinary lines."

Much of public health epidemiological research and interventions has focused on individual-level factors in understanding the cause of between-population differences in disease rates and have promoted interventions that rely on change emerging from individual-level behavioral choices. (Berkman 2004; Diez Roux 2004). Cohen and Syme (1985) explain, "an individual perspective…addresses the question of why one person gets sick while another person does not. A social perspective addresses the question of why one group or aggregation has a higher rate of disease than another…interventions can be viewed from both perspectives…the issue is not whether one approach is better than another but the usefulness of different approaches depending on their purpose."

Krieger (1994) discusses the limitations of what she calls "biomedical individualism" and challenges the current rigid distinction between individual and group-level analyses. She notes that there are health effects of groups that cannot be reduced to individual attributes. Corin (1994) states that individual health behavior cannot be fully understood unless the social and cultural context in which it is embedded is understood. The social context for studying the health behavior of groups is complex, dynamic, and needs to utilize diverse methods. Therefore, analyses of group behavior involves more than simply aggregating or averaging individual measures, or gathering observational data, or using multiple regression methods to control for individual-level confounding variables. When a determinant of health at the societal or group level of analysis is not confirmed as a risk factor in studies at the individual level of analysis, the societal finding is labeled an "ecological fallacy."

The health dynamics of populations or groups may involve factors that account for only a small part of individual variation in health and may escape detection. On the other hand, factors responsible for major differences in populations or groups may be so common that they go undetected in studies of individuals (Wilkinson 1996). The influence of social factors shared by most everyone in a population or group can only be detected by comparing different populations or groups. Important explanations for health differences between individuals do not explain differences within or between populations or groups.

Different levels of analyses produce different pictures of the determinants of health and different pictures of the effectiveness of health interventions (Jepson et al. 2010). Studies of individuals lead to attempts to distinguish between people with and without some disease or social problem who all belong to the same population or social group. Comparisons of different groups with and without the same disease or social problem help to identify shared and unshared characteristics common to the problem, or help to identify common mechanisms by which the same problem is generated or prevented from occurring across different social and cultural contexts.

1.8.1 Interventions to Reduce Disparities

Rust and Cooper (2007) state that very few interventional studies have demonstrated significant reductions in health disparities. While there is no best literature on quality of improvement and health promotion, none of the research to date has had an impact on reducing health disparities. Rust and Cooper offer 12 strategies that they say could help improve disparities research. First, there is a need to conduct disparities research in settings that serve high-disparity communities. A second strategy would involve more investigators from diverse groups who have a sensitivity to bias or blinders and who are racially and culturally representative of the population or group being studied. Third, a shared partnership of power and money and sharing data and its interpretation would also produce a greater commitment to the research on a long-term basis. Four, changing the system has been found to improve disparities-relevant services, that is paying attention to processes of care can have an effect on disparities. Five, interventions need to be conducted in the community context where patients live. Six, interventions to reduce disparities must move to the population level and address multiple factors relating to disparities. Seven, interventions should be broader than focusing on a single disease. Co-morbidities abound in high-disparity populations. Eight, traditional experimental study designs test only one intervention. No single intervention is likely to

Table 1.4 Estimates of burden of disease for those health conditions that had a higher incidence or prevalence in South Texas than in the rest of Texas

Health status indicator	South Texas incidence/ prevalence per 100,000 population	Incidence/prevalence difference between South Texas and the rest of Texas, per 100,000 population
Obesity (adult)	29,500.0	4500.0
Diabetes	9,100.0	1700.0
Chlamydia	345.0	34.3
Other birth defects	13.0–221.0	5.1–48.1
Neural tube defects	98.0	32.0
Cervical cancer	11.5	1.4
Liver cancer	10.2	3.5
Tuberculosis	8.6	1.7
Stomach cancer	8.6	1.6
Leukemia (child and adolescent)	5.6	0.9
Gallbladder cancer	1.5	0.5
Pesticide poisoning	1.2	0.3

Source Ramiriz et al. (2013, p. 144)

make a difference in reducing health disparities. Nine, a static unchanging intervention is poorly suited to dynamic environments and should be held constant throughout the study. Ten, disparities research needs a rapid-change model with feedback loops. Eleven, optimal study design is not only driven by research vigor but also by a sense of partnership with communities. Twelve, sometimes interventions that are tested in real-world settings may not be sustainable when grant funding is withdrawn. Ultimately real-world reductions in health disparities require interventions that are not only effective, but replicable and sustainable.

Rust and Cooper (2007) point out that these strategies may come with costs, but the bulk of research to date has not reduced disparities especially at the community and population levels. Diez Roux (2008) notes that there needs to be new directions in the investigation of multilevel determinants in disparity research such as improving the measurement of group-level constructs, examine contexts other than neighborhoods, analyze data from natural experiments, develop methodological approaches that examine dependencies between groups and their sources and allow for and explore reciprocal relations and feedback loops between individuals and contexts. Diez Roux (2008) notes that while the contribution of multilevel analysis has promoted multilevel thinking and the development and testing of multilevel questions in epidemiology, we must guard against the multilevel approach not becoming an end in itself but rather as a tool to understand, intervene in, and change, health disparities.

A recent review of the incidence or prevalence of health conditions in South Texas in comparison with Texas point out 13 health status indicators that contribute the most to the burden of disease in Texas border counties and communities (Ramiriz et al. 2013). Table 1.4 shows the extent to which each of 13 health status indicators are disparate from the Texas population.

The prevalence of adult obesity and diabetes in South Texas are almost twice that for the state as a whole. Chlamydia in South Texas is about ten times the rate for the entire state. Other birth defects, especially neural tube defects are two to three times as frequent in South Texas compared to the state as a whole. Several types of cancer, especially cervical, liver, stomach, leukemia, and gallbladder are more frequent in the South Texas border compared to the state. Tuberculosis and pesticide poisoning are also more frequent in South Texas than in Texas as a whole.

Table 1.5 shows the comparisons of 28 health status indicators from South Texas to Texas as a whole, from South Texas to the U.S. as a whole, to comparing Hispanics with non-Hispanics in South Texas, to comparing Hispanics in South Texas to Hispanics in Texas as a whole. In all comparisons the highest rates for tuberculosis, liver cancer, and adult obesity are in South Texas. Chlamydia, cervical cancer, gallbladder cancer, neural tube defects and diabetes have the highest rates in three of the comparisons. Stomach cancer, leukemia, and birth defects, have the highest rates in two of the comparisons. The lack of data prohibits accurate comparisons to be made for the remaining health status indicators.

It is also instructive to note in Table 1.5 those health status indicators that have low rates in South Texas compared to the whole of Texas or the U.S. Breast cancer, colorectal cancer, prostate cancer, lung cancer, motor vehicle crash mortality, and suicide are all low compared to Texas and the U.S.

Many of these disparities may be associated with a higher percentage of persons with no health insurance in South Texas compared to the rest of Texas. An estimated one-third of the South Texas population has no health insurance— a barrier in receiving preventive care or treatment for health conditions (Ramiriz et al. 1995).

Ramiriz et al. (2013) made several recommendations based on their review of disparities. Since obesity has the greatest impact on South Texas of all of the health conditions examined, prevention research should focus on obesity and diabetes. Obesity is especially important because it is a risk for diabetes and also associated with some cancers and cardiovascular disease, and some birth defects. Two modifiable behaviors affecting obesity are insufficient physical activity and poor nutrition; these also should be the focus of intervention research in South Texas.

1.8.2   Examples of Gaps and Deficiencies in Disparity Research Along the U.S.-Mexico Border Smoking Cessation

The leading causes of morbidity and mortality among Hispanics living in the U.S. are smoking related, specifically cardiovascular disease and lung cancer. Evidence suggests that the prevalence of smoking in this population will increase as Hispanics become more acculturated (Webb et al. 2010). Yet, of 12 intervention

Table 1.5 Comparison of whether South Texas has a higher or lower rate than the rest of Texas or nationwide as well as whether Hispanics have a higher or lower rate than non-Hispanic whites in South Texas for each health indicator

Health status indicator	South Texas, compared with the rest of Texas	South Texas, compared with the nation	South Texas Hispanics, compared with non-Hispanic whites in South Texas	South Texas Hispanics, compared with Hispanics in the rest of Texas
Tuberculosis	Higher	Higher	Higher	Higher
HIV/AIDS	Lower	- - - -	Higher	Lower
Syphilis	Lower	- - - -	Higher	Lower
Chlamydia	Higher	- - - -	Higher	Higher
Gonorrhea	Lower	- - - -	Higher	Higher
Breast cancer	Lower	Lower	Lower	Higher
Cervical cancer	Higher	Higher	Higher	*
Colorectal cancer	Lower	Lower	Lower	Higher
Prostate cancer	Lower	Lower	Lower	Lower
Lung cancer	Lower	Lower	Lower	*
Liver cancer	Higher	Higher	Higher	Higher
Stomach cancer	Higher	*	Higher	*
Gallbladder cancer	Higher	Higher	Higher	*
Leukemia	Higher	Higher	*	*
Neural tube defects	Higher	- - - -	Higher	Higher
Oral clefts	*	- - - -	*	*
Other birth defects	Higher	Higher	*	*
Infant mortality	Lower	- - - -	*	*
Diabetes	Higher	Higher	*	Higher
Heart disease mortality	Lower	- - - -	*	Higher
Cerebrovascular disease mortality	Lower	- - - -	*	*
Asthma (adult)	*	*	*	*
Obesity (adult)	Higher	Higher	Higher	Higher
Childhood lead poisoning	*	- - - -	Higher	*
Pesticide poisoning	Higher	- - - -	*	Higher
Motor vehicle crash mortality	Lower	- - - -	Lower	Lower
Homicide	*	*	Higher	Lower
Suicide	Lower	Lower	Lower	*

Source Ramiriz et al. (2013, p. 141)
*Cells left blank denote similar rates between the two groups being compared
Dotted line means that nationwide data were not available to make the comparison between South Texas and the nation

studies on smoking cessation that emerged since 1991 from a literature review and meta-analysis, only three were community-based interventions (Webb et al. 2010). While the strengths of these studies were their focus on a culturally specific approach, and the inclusion of a behavioral component, they were limited by high attrition, lack of comparison groups, short follow-up periods, unmatched treatment conditions, restricted age ranges, and nonrepresentative samples.

Future research should address these methodological limitations exploring the direct relationship between intervention and smoking status, as well as the interactive and mediating relationships between smoking and cultural variables. It is important that intervention designs recognize the significant heterogeneity among Hispanics that often have different language patterns and values. Multi-site interventions with large and representative samples also increase the generalizability of findings. Future research and intervention studies should also consider the influence of acculturation, which has been shown to be related to tobacco initiation and treatment outcomes.

Reducing tobacco smoking can reduce morbidity and mortality, therefore future research and intervention activities have the potential of significantly impacting the health of border residents as well as Hispanics in the general U.S. population.

1.8.2.1 Preventing and Controlling Tuberculosis

Performance of TB control programs among the U.S.-Mexico binational population has not been characterized adequately in terms of prevention and treatment interventions because program evaluation requires sharing performance indicators especially: (1) targeted testing of specific high risk groups including persons with HIV infections and diabetes, immigrants, and medically underserved persons; (2) cooperation to strengthen diagnostic capabilities in Mexican border states, and (3) improved contact tracing by enhancing knowledge of social patterns of binational tracings and by developing a common contact protocol for the U.S. and Mexico (Lobato et al. 2001).

A Work Group Report (Lobato et al. 2001) proposed a multilevel approach to intervention in TB prevention and control. The Centers for Disease Control would work with state and local TB control programs and collaborate with public health and social scientists to develop and evaluate innovative methods for tracing, testing, and treating contacts of binational patients. Studies could then compare new strategies with past practices.

1.8.2.2 Knowledge-Action Gap in Diabetes

Type 2 diabetes (DM2) is the first cause of death in Mexico and the third leading cause in the U.S. A recent prevalence study that focused on a representative binational border population sample and used a common methodology found that 15 % of the U.S.-Mexico border population aged 18 years and older were affected by DM2 and 14 % were in the pre-diabetic stage (Cerqueira 2010). Evidence points to the need to create supportive environments for active lifestyles, increase access to healthy and affordable foods, improve outreach and access to quality health services, continue research to ascertain effective interventions, and increase surveillance along the border using a common methodology. Diabetes is a community issue (Ingram et al. 2005). There is a need to identify elements of successful intervention programs such as using promotoras in outreach and education and community partnerships (Ingram et al. 2005).

1.8.2.3 HIV Prevention

Organista et al. (2004) reviewed and critiqued the HIV prevention outcome literature on Mexican migrants including U.S.-Mexico border inhabitants to identify gaps and recommend future research directions. They pointed to three overlapping complex approaches used to guide HIV prevention research. The first and predominant paradigm has been the behavioral approach based on theories of individual psychology that links HIV transmission primarily to behavioral and cognitive factors and co-factors such as drug use. A second approach builds on the first including social and cultural contexts that influence individual and group risk-related behaviors. A third approach focuses on structural, environmental, and social change issues. The authors point out that future research, service, and policy could be advanced if all three approaches were integrated.

Today, HIV prevention for Mexican migrants and related groups consists primarily of minimal and inconsistent HIV/AIDS education, condom promotion and distribution, HIV testing and counseling, and support groups for affected individuals. For example, Moyer et al. (2008), found that only 38 % of injection drug users in Tijuana and 30 % in Ciudad Juarez had ever had an HIV test. Community-based organizations that provide health and social services have been found to be more effective in reaching Latinos than federal and state agencies because of their greater number of bilingual staff, volunteers, and culturally sensitive approaches to service delivery. While community-based interventions designed to improve knowledge of HIV transmissions are effective this approach is embedded in the individual cognitive model and does not address larger contextual aspects of HIV risk such as migration-related prostitution. Along the U.S.-Mexico border regional dynamics such as the drug and sex trade industries, tourism, transnationalism, and blurred sexual boundaries can result in significant HIV infections.

There is a need to increase our understanding of HIV risk, with an emphasis on sexuality and the ways that sex practices and beliefs vary across subgroups of migrants and border residents, and across different social, cultural, and relational contexts. Randomized controlled trends are difficult to implement with certain populations, but quasi-experimental research designs and mixed methods can be very useful. There is a need for conducting broader and more rigorous replications and/or modifications to better fit local research settings and subgroups of border migrants.

1.8.2.4 Environmental Issues

The North American Free Trade Agreement (NAFTA) and the presence of maquiladoras have intensified long-standing concerns about environmental health and hazardous waste issues along the U.S.-Mexico border. There are significant gaps in information about environmental quality. Current environmental quality monitoring focuses on air quality and surface water quality near large urban centers, but hazardous waste is not addressed (Carter et al. 1996). Specifically, environmental levels of pesticides and possible human exposure routes are not being targeted. Also, colonias' sources of water and their levels of hazardous wastes need monitoring (Southwest Center for Environmental Research and Policy 2012).

Data gaps are a great problem because baseline information is necessary to better control and improve the identification of chemically induced diseases. To identify environmental health problems in the border region, the baseline incidence of disease must be determined in both U.S. and Mexican states. The influence of nutrition on chemical toxicity needs investigation. In the U.S. the border region is populated by a substantially lower socioeconomic class than in the rest of the country, a characteristic that is often limited to a higher incidence of nutritional deficiencies and more frequent exposure to infectious diseases. The incidence of lupus and the role of chemicals in its development needs investigation. Finally, analysis is needed of the data being generated at the border. Several state and federal agencies have established programs to analyze chemicals in air, water, and soil, but there are no efforts to analyze the data for trends, source of hazardous waste, or profiles of chemical waste. More targeted research is needed to evaluate the health impact of various wastes and waste treatment processes.

A U.S.-Mexico workshop was held to discuss many of the above issues. Recommendations were made, however, it was unclear to whom the recommendations should be directed (Carter et al. 1996). While there is heightened awareness of the environmental problems along the border and the data gaps that exist, progress is limited because it is undetermined who should take the lead, and how, and by whom, accountability will be assumed for solving these binational problems.

1.8.2.5 Mental Health

Discriminatory experiences have been found to be related to poor mental health outcomes and negative life changes among marginalized communities in the United States. Many socioeconomic and environmental conditions negatively influence the mental health of borderlanders including poverty, the lack of resources, drug trafficking, violence and immigration risks (Flores and Kaplan 2009). There is a paucity of studies of the mental health of borderlanders. Focus groups among Mexican Americans living along the southern border of Texas identified the lack of resources, knowledge about the causes and treatment for mental health problems, the importance of kinship among Hispanics, and the lack of providers who understood their needs as several key problems. Indicators of mental health issues encountered by borderlanders have been extracted from some U.S. prevalence studies that address the mental health of Latinos. In general, U.S.-born Latinos are at significantly higher risk for most psychiatric disorders compared to Latino immigrants and non-Latino whites. Traditional cultural practices have been suggested as a protective factor for Latino immigrants.

Cultural adaptations of evidence-based practices are necessary for treatment interventions to meet the needs of individuals, families, and communities, to impact treatment engagement, and to improve treatment outcomes. Even when borderlanders suffer from mental health problems they may not be able to access treatment due to their immigration status, fear, or knowledge of, and access to, resources. Furthermore, mental health care may not be a priority when individuals and families are faced with homelessness, poverty, hunger, violence and other problems related to daily survival. A significant amount of literature has pointed out that cultural values, language and level of acculturation are key variables in health care professionals and borderlanders experiencing biculturalism as the best model for positive mental health outcomes.

1.8.3 How Far Have We Come in Reducing Health Disparities in the U.S.?

In 2010 the Institute of Medicine (IOM) sponsored a workshop to assess the progress that had been made in the U.S. in reducing health disparities since the IOM and Surgeon General released several reports on disparities in 2000 (U.S. Dept. HHS 2005, 2011; Institute of Medicine 2001; Smedley et al. 2003).

Findings show that over the past decade no significant change in disparities had occurred for at least 70 % of the leading indicator objectives. The groups seeing the fewest advances were American Indians and Alaska Natives. Life expectancy has steadily increased since 1970, but major disparities remain. African American males have the shortest life expectancy of all groups. HIV infection/AIDS is another area in which large discrepancies exist, especially among African American men who are at high risk of dying from HIV infection (Koh et al. 2010).

Mortality rates due to coronary heart disease were met for all groups except African Americans, who have higher mortality rates from coronary heart disease than other groups. The gap between African Americans and the group with the lowest rates (Asians) needs to be narrowed (Institute of Medicine 2012).

The gap between the group with the highest rate of mammography screening (whites) and the group with the lowest (Latinos) has narrowed, however the rates for poor women are low compared to those for middle and high-income women.

Racial/ethnic disparities in childhood vaccination rates have narrowed significantly since the mid-1990s, but the same narrowing in adult immunization rates has not occurred.

The trend of increased rates of obesity in the U.S. is worsening especially among Blacks and Mexican-Americans of both sexes. Childhood obesity has continually increased from the 1970s to 2004. Disproportionate rates of childhood obesity exist across the U.S. with southern states having the highest rates. Obesity is an example of a disparity that can be prevented.

Latinos are the population least likely to be insured; this group is the least insured among all racial and ethnic groups in Massachusetts even after the passage of health reform legislation in that state.

Anne Beal, President of the Aetna Foundation, outlined the evolution of health disparities research and summed up progress stating "all disparities are local" (Institute of Medicine 2012, pp. 75–78). Although national data are useful in moving to evidence-based action plans, what is needed are more localized and focused action plans. Research describing disparities is not needed. What is needed are evidence-based action plans, what Braveman et al. (2004), Braveman (2006) has called "intervention research." Beal said that one of the challenges to creating an evidence-based action plan is that it requires a fresh approach to research. Reductionistic approaches will not work for health disparities. No single factor can be considered the root cause of disparities. Beal noted that national data can be useful in providing direction, local data are needed to determine appropriate interventions.

1.9 The Border Region as a Social System

The binational region shared by Mexico and the United States and its inhabitants is a social system. The region shares environmental, social, economic, cultural and health characteristics while retaining national sovereignty and different legal, political, and health systems, and public policies. Mexico and the United States are both independent and interdependent social systems. The actions and inactions of inhabitants on one side of the border have repercussions for inhabitants on the other side. The nature of this interrelationship is dynamic, complex, and constantly challenged by inadequate economic resources, changing politics, cultural and language differences and population growth.

A social system has many different levels of organization. In the case of Mexico and the U.S. the major levels are national, regional, state, county, and municipal. Ranging from the municipal level to the national level, each level is an incremental increase in social complexity. No level alone can completely explain the phenomenon occurring at that level, since all levels are interrelated. For example, factors at the national and regional levels are involved in the functioning of Mexican and U.S. communities. Each level explains only part of a total social system; for example, behavior at a higher or more complex level cannot be predicted from behavior at a lower level (Mabry et al. 2008).

The goal of a social system is to achieve and maintain a balance between its parts so that it functions with relative cohesion and works constructively with other social systems. Activities that are defined as problems upset the cohesion or balance of a social system. Problem-solving and intervention is initiated to restore a sense of balance or equilibrium to an unbalanced one. The task of the problem solver is to learn how the system operates, especially what factors help it function in a positive manner, and assist with bringing about positive change. It is difficult, if not impossible to introduce change to one part of a system without affecting all parts of the system. The challenge is to learn what facilitates and inhibits balance in a social system with the intention of minimizing or controlling them so that the system can be enhanced and function in a preferred way (Bruhn and Rebach 2007).

A systems approach to solving and preventing border health problems has several advantages: (1) it can focus on several related problems simultaneously; (2) it identifies relationships where the cost of intervention is lowest and the effectiveness of intervention is highest; (3) it shifts the emphasis from quick-fix solutions to sustainable ones; (4) it includes options in solutions to adapt to change; (5) it helps maintain the integrity of complexity of a living system. Border health problems are simultaneously local and national; therefore, interventions at only one level will not bring about lasting solutions to problems (Bruhn and Rebach 2007). For example, an educational and outreach intervention to positively impact self-management behaviors for diabetes will be more sustainable and successful if it involves a consortium of providers at the community and county levels and an academic partner who provides technical assistance and objective evaluation (Ingram et al. 2005).

An example of the social systems approach is the U.S.-Mexico Border Diabetes Prevention and Control Project prevalence study (Cerqueira 2010). This study considered the U.S.-Mexico border area as an integral unit. Border counties and communities share more similarities among themselves than they do with their respective countries, especially in the case of U.S.-Mexico sister cities. This study used a representative binational border sample and a common methodology. The project has demonstrated the feasibility of effective, binational, interinstitutional, multi-disciplinary teamwork to achieve the common good of diabetes prevention and control.

1.9.1 Meso Level Interventions

The meso level has been a common intervention point in border health initiatives. People experience society in interaction with others at the meso level in a variety of organizations and social networks such as communities, organizations, neighborhoods, gangs, clubs, public agencies, corporate boards, and businesses. It is through these meso level structures that we find our identities and meet a variety of needs beyond those of the individual and family. These mediating structures link the macro and micro levels of a society. It is through the meso level that we can best intervene to solve problems. The meso level provides grassroots understanding and data about the reality of everyday life. Indeed, to effect change in border health problems, there must be a buy-in and active support from citizens on both sides of the border. This is a challenge because culturally the same problem may be perceived differently and/or economic and survival needs may give the same problem different priorities. Facilitators of communication such as community health workers or *promotoras* have been found to successfully serve as "bridges" between community members and health care services (CDC Workgroup 2001). An emerging body of literature appears to support the unique role of the community worker and advocates in strengthening existing community networks for care, providing community members with support, education, and facilitating access to care (CDC Division of Diabetes Translation 2011; Steinfelt 2005; Balcazar et al. 2009a, b; Elder et al. 2009; Hunter et al. 2004; Lara 1998; Ford et al. 1998; Brandon 1997).

Promotoras have been effective in providing appropriate context for interventions in a wide range of problems from hypertension control (Balcazar et al. 2009a, b), comprehensive preventive care (Hunter et al. 2004), depression (Waitzkin et al. 2011) to improving pesticide safety (Forster-Cox et al. 2007). The *promotoras* is a meso level mechanism to create behavior change among individuals and families. The *promotoras*, however, are unlikely to effect significant systemic changes without assistance from macro level bureaucracies and agencies that shape health policy and allocate resources.

1.9.2   Data in the Intervention Process

1.9.2.1   Level of Analysis/Establishing a Need to Intervene

Interventions are only as effective as the data used to plan them. Although the U.S. and Mexico are two different geopolitical systems, the components or elements that make up the systems, e.g., national, regional, states, municipios, are similar. Therefore, there is some degree of comparability between, for example, a U.S. border community and a Mexican municipios. Similarly, the 14 sister cities are both distinct social systems but together form a bi-cultural, geopolitical system unique to themselves. Understanding the differences and commonalities of the different levels of analysis is key to cross border interventions. For example, out of the 46 Mexican National Health Indicators and 25 United States Healthy Gente objectives there are 20 common measures. These represent priority areas for actions on health issues in the border region. However, differences in the national organization of health care service and data availability program objectives for both sides of the border are defined and refined by each county, state, or community (U.S.–Mexico Border Health Commission, Healthy Border 2010a, b). While culturally unique interventions are needed and respected, real progress will come in the future from binational interventions, especially those at the community/municipios level of analysis (Cerqueira 2009). Differences in data definitions and availability will need to be overcome and a common binational data collection and retrieval bank will need to be established if creditable, comparable, and consistent information for planning and implementing interventions is to occur.

A common level of analysis used in intervention programs to date has been those implemented at the community/municipios level. At the community level it is usually easier to access information from subjects and involve them in establishing the need for an intervention as well as to implement programs and activities that will directly translate to practice.

1.9.3 The Intervention Plan

After data has shown a need for an intervention it is useful to solicit the involvement of private and public collaborators and partners in planning the interventions to insure that the plan will be culturally appropriate, meet needs, and be sustainable. Intervention plans usually falter if there is no clear goal at the onset and the objectives and strategies for reaching the goal are not clear to all parties involved. If there is no clearly agreed upon buy-into the plan by all constituents it is likely the plan will be plagued with setbacks and will be unsustainable, when and if, it is completed. A good intervention plan needs to be flexible, anticipate and plan for change, yet not be too rigid about meeting the intended goal.

1.9.4 Baseline Data

Many interventions become scientifically unsound if they do not use baseline data for planning an intervention. Ideally, the baseline data should include objective measures, but also include subjective data such as those from focus groups, interviews, and surveys as well. Data collected in the course of carrying out the intervention should be comparable to that in the baseline. In the case of a binational intervention the variables and their meanings and measurements should be agreed upon if the baseline is to be common to both cultures.

1.9.5 Intervention Data

An intervention should be comprehensive in its measurements of the scope of its impact. As such the evaluation of an intervention needs to collect both process data and program data. Program data will provide evidence of the extent the intervention met its goal. Process data provides evidence the intervention plan was executed according to plan with minimal bias and subject drop-out. Both levels of data are needed if the intervention is to be replicated with improvements. Both program and process data are important in bicultural interventions when the subtleties of language and culture can be factors in the success or failure of an intervention.

1.9.6 Follow-Up Data

Some follow-up data are needed to gain insight into the sustainability of interventions. This is a special challenge for interventions on the U.S.-Mexico border where geographical mobility and anonymity are features of daily life. Short-term follow-up of less than six months is not an unreasonable goal, long-term follow-ups of 1 year or longer are a challenge. Working at the community level enables follow-ups as it is more likely *promotoras* would be able to learn and access the social networks of small communities. Follow-ups need to be part of the recruitment of participants for any intervention, especially a commitment of their willingness to provide brief access to them.

1.9.7 Translation to Practice

Binational, bicultural interventions are especially challenged to be practical, useful, and to fit into one's culture as comfortably as possible if follow through and lifestyle changes are a goal. Indeed, any intervention threatens one's values and their prioritization in one's life. Part of the intervention could incorporate the opportunity to discuss the impact of an intervention on one's self, family and extended family. This would also provide the opportunity for interveners to learn more about the personal and familial aspects of health behavior change and provide insights about how border residents can be more fully engaged in making health choices.

1.9.8 Sharing Data

There is a need to replicate well-designed intervention studies to improve generalizability such as the use of *promotoras*, and evaluate and compare various intervention models at different levels of analysis. More intervention studies need to be designed cross-culturally so that partnerships and shared resources can be used to enhance sustainability on both sides of the border. Border centers of excellence can facilitate the establishment of shared databases to reduce duplication, costs, and personnel and initiate projects that will build on the capacity of successful models.

1.10 Summary

The U.S.-Mexico border region presents many challenges to the typical model of intervention in public health. A social systems approach which links individual, group, and population levels of data seems appropriate for understanding how and why micro and macro factors interact to produce positive and negative health effects. A systems approach provides a holistic understanding of risks and protective factors that give rise to certain health behaviors. Moreover, a systems approach provides insights into how health interventions can be effective in creating behavioral change and increase sustainability.

The social systems approach embraces cultural uniqueness and differences, and as such, is a useful model for health interventions along the U.S.-Mexico border. Many interventions have fallen short of the usual process followed in intervention studies, hence, generalizability and reproducibility are compromised. Future data needs include sharing databases and establishing collaborations so that more interventions can be carried out with greater scientific rigor and yield stronger applications to practice.

The 2012 Health Care Disparities Report from the Department of Health and Human Services stated the need to accelerate programs if we are to achieve higher quality and equitable health care. Health care and access are suboptimal, especially for minority and low-income groups. Overall quality is improving, access is getting worse and disparities are not changing. We need continued improvements in the quality of diabetes care, maternal and child health, disparities in cancer care, and the quality of care especially in the Southern states (U.S. Dept. of HHS 2013).

References

Adler, N., & Newman, K. (2002). Socioeconomic disparities in health: Pathways and policies. *Health Affairs, 21*(2), 60–76.

Adler, N. E., & Rehkopf, D. H. (2008). U.S. disparities in health: Descriptions, causes and mechanisms. *Annual Review of Public Health, 29*, 235–252.

Balcazar, H., Alvarado, M., Fulwood, R., Pedregon, V., & Cantu, F. (2009a). A promotora de salud model for addressing cardiovascular disease risk factors in the U.S.-Mexico Border Region. *Preventing Chronic Diesase, 6*(1), 02.

Balcazar, H. G., Byrd, T. L., Ortiz, M., Tondapu, S. R., & Chavez, M. (2009b). A randomized community intervention to improve hypertension control among Mexican Americans: Using the promotoras de salud community outreach model. *Journal of Health Care for the Poor and Underserved, 20*(4), 1079–1094.

Bastida, E. (2001). Kinship ties of Mexican migrant women on the United States/Mexico border. *Journal of Comparative Family Studies, 32*(4), 549–569.

Bastida, E., Brown, H. S., & Pagan, J. A. (2008). Persistent disparities in the use of health care along the U.S.-Mexico border: An ecological perspective. *American Journal of Public Health, 98*(11), 1987–1995.

Bergner, M., & Rothman, M. L. (1987). Health status measures: An overview and guide for selection. *Annual Review of Public Health, 8*, 191–210.

Berkman, L. F. (2004). Introduction: Seeing the forest and the trees—From observation to experiments in social epidemiology. *Epidemiological Reviews, 26*(1), 2–6.

Bilheimer, L. T., & Sisk, J. E. (2008). Collecting adequate data on racial and ethnic disparities in health: The challenges continue. *Health Affairs, 27*(2), 383–391.

Bleich, S. N., Jarlenski, M. P., Bell, C. N., & LaVeist, T. A. (2012). Health inequalities: Trends, progress and policy. *Annual Review of Public Health, 33*, 7–40.

Brandon, J. E. (1997). Health promotion efforts along the U.S.-Mexico border. In J. G. Bruhn & J. E. Brandon (Eds.), *Border health: Challenges for the United States and Mexico* (pp. 163–179). New York: Garland Publishing Inc.

Braveman, P. (2006). Health disparities and health equity: Concepts and measurement. *Annual Review of Public Health, 27*, 167–194.

Braveman, P. A., Egerter, S. A., Cubbin, C., & Marchi, K. S. (2004). An approach to studying social disparities in health and health care. *American Journal of Public Health, 94*(12), 2139–2148.

Braveman, P., Egerter, S., & Williams, D. R. (2011). The social determinants of health: Coming of age. *Annual Review of Public Health, 32*, 381–398.

Bruhn, J. G. (1997). Health: Its meaning and expression. In J. G. Bruhn & J. E. Brandon (Eds.), *Border health: Challenges for the United States and Mexico* (pp. 13–36). New York: Garland Publishing Inc.

Bruhn, J. G. (2009). *The group effect: Social cohesion and health outcomes.* New York: Springer.

Bruhn, J. G., & Rebach, H. M. (2007). *Sociological practice: Intervention and social change.* New York: Springer.

Byrd, W. M., & Clayton, L. A. (2003). Racial and ethnic disparities in health care: A background and history. In B. Smedley, A. Y. Stith, & A. R. Nelson (Eds.), *Unequal treatment: Confronting racial and ethnic disparities in health care* (pp. 455–527). Washington, DC: Institute of Medicine, The National Academies Press.

Byrd, T. L., & Law, J. G. (2009). Cross-border utilization of health care services by United States residents living near the Mexican border. *Revista Panamericana de Salud Publica, 26*(2), 95–100.

Campbell, D. (1974). Downward causation in hierarchically organized biological systems. In F. J. Ayala & T. Dobzhansky (Eds.), *Studies in the philosophy of biology: Reduction and related problems* (pp. 179–186). Berkeley, CA: University of California Press.

Carter, D. E., Pena, C., Varady, R., & Suk, W. A. (1996). Environmental health and hazardous waste issues related to the U.S.-Mexico border. *Environmental Health Perspectives, 104*, 590–594.

Carter-Pokras, O., & Baquet, C. (2002). What is a health disparity? *Public Health Reports, 117*(5), 426–434.

CDC Division of Diabetes Translation and Division of Adult and Community Health (2011). Community Health Worker and Promotora de Salud Workgroup Members. Community Health Workers/Promotoras de Salud: Critical Connections in Communities. Retrieved January 15, 2011 from http://www.cdc.gov/diabetes/projects/comm.htm

CDC Workgroup (2001). Community Health Workers. http://www.cdc.gov/diabetes/projects/comm.htm

Cerqueira, M. T. (2009). Center of Excellence, Pan American Health Organization (PAHO), U.S.-Mexico Border Office. www.borderhealth.org/border_models_of_excellence.php?curr=bhc_initiatives.Retrieved January, 25 2011.

Cerqueira, M. T. (2010). Bridging the knowledge-action gap in diabetes along the U.S.-Mexico border. *Revista Panamericana de Salud Publica/Pan American Journal of Public Health, 28*(3), 139–140.

Chavez, L. R., Cornelius, W. A., & Jones, O. W. (1985). Mexican immigrants and the utilization of U.S. health services: The case of San Diego. *Social Science in Medicine, 21*(1), 93–102.

Cohen, S., & Syme, S. L. (1985). *Social support and health* (p. 19). New York: Academic Press.

Corin, E. (1994). The social and cultural matrix of health and disease. In R. G. Evans, M. L. Barer, & T. R. Marmor (Eds.), *Why are some people healthy and others not? The determinants of health of populations* (pp. 93–132). New York: Walter de Gruyter.

Dakubo, C. Y. (2010). *Ecosystems and human health.* New York: Springer.

Dear, M. (2013). *Why walls won't work: Repairing the U.S.- Mexico divide.* New York: Oxford University Press.

Diez Roux, A. V. (2004). The study of group-level factors in epidemiology: Rethinking variables, study designs, and analytical approaches. *Epidemiologic Reviews, 26*(1), 104–111.

Diez Roux, A. V. (2008). Next steps in understanding the multilevel determinants of health. *Journal of Epidemiology and Community Health, 62*(11), 957–959.

Diez Roux, A. V. (2011). Complex systems thinking and current impasses in health disparities research. *American Journal of Public Health, 101*(9), 1627–1634.

Diez Roux, A. V. (2012). Conceptual approaches to the study of health disparities. *Annual Review of Public Health, 33*, 41–58.

Elder, J. P., Ayala, G. X., Parra-Medina, D., & Talavera, G. A. (2009). Health communication in the Latino community: Issues and approaches. *Annual Review of Public Health, 30*, 227–251.

Environmental Protection Agency (EPA) (2011). U.S.-Mexico Border. Accessed at http://www.epa.gov/SoCal/border.html

Flores, L., & Kaplan, A. (Eds.). (2009). *Addressing the mental health problems of border and immigrant youth.* Los Angeles, CA: National Center for Child Traumatic Stress.

Ford, L. A., Barnes, M. D., Crabtree, R. D., & Fairbanks, J. (1998). Boundary spanners: Las promotoras in the borderlands. In J. G. Power & T. Byrd (Eds.), *U.S.-Mexico border health: Issues for regional and migrant populations* (pp. 141–164). Thousand Oaks, CA: Sage.

Forster-Cox, S. C., Mangadu, T., Jacquez, B., & Corona, A. (2007). The effectiveness of the promotora (Community Health Worker) model of intervention for improving pesticide safety in U.S./Mexico border homes. *Californian Journal of Health Promotion, 5*(1), 62–75.

Freimuth, V. S., & Quinn, S. C. (2004). The contributions of health communication to eliminating health disparities. *American Journal of Public Health, 94*(12), 2053–2055.

Ganster, P., & Lorey, D. E. (2008). *The U.S.-Mexico border in the 21st century* (2nd ed.). Lanham, MD: Rowman & Littlefield Pub.

Gehlert, S., Sohmer, D., Sacks, T., Mininger, C., McClintock, M., & Olopade, O. (2008). Targeting health disparities: A model linking upstream determinants to downstream interventions. *Health Affairs, 27*(2), 339–349.

Gerber, J. (2009). *Developing the U.S.-Mexico border region for a prosperous and secure relationship: Human and physical infrastructure along the U.S. border with Mexico.* Houston, TX: Institute for Public Policy, Rice University.

Gibbons, M. C. (2005). A historical overview of health disparities and the potential of ehealth solutions. *Journal of Internet Research, 7*(5), e50.

Glanz, K., & Bishop, D. B. (2010). The role of behavioral science theory in development and implementation of public health interventions. *Annual Review of Public Health, 31*, 399–418.

Glasgow, R. E., Vogt, T. M., & Boles, S. M. (1999). Evaluating the public health impact of health promotion interventions: The RE-AIM framework. *American Journal of Public Health, 89*, 1322–1327.

Glasgow, R. E., Klesges, L. M., Dzewaltowski, D. A., Bull, S. S., & Estrabrooks, P. (2004). The future of health behavior change research: What is needed to improve translation of research into health promotion practice. *Annals of Behavioral Medicine, 27*(1), 3–12.

Glass, T. A. (2000). Psychosocial intervention. In L. Berkman & I. Kawachi (Eds.), *Social epidemiology* (pp. 267–305). New York: Oxford University Press.

Good Neighbor Environmental Board (GNEB) & Environmental Advisors Across Borders. (2010). *Blueprint for action on the U.S.-Mexico border.* Thirteenth Report of the Good Neighbor Environmental Board to the President and Congress of the United States, June 2010.

Herbert, P. L., Sisk, J. E., & Howell, E. A. (2008). When does a difference become a disparity? Conceptualizing racial and ethnic disparities in health. *Health Affairs, 27*(2), 374–382.

Homedes, N., & Ugalde, A. (2003). Globalization and health at the United States-Mexico border. *American Journal of Public Health, 93*(12), 2016–2022.

Homedes, N. & Ugalde, A. (2009). Shaping health reform for the U.S.-Mexico border region. *Texas Business Review, October,* 1–5.

Hunter, J. B., de Zapien, J. G., Papenfuss, M., Fernandez, M. L., Meister, J., & Giuliano, A. R. (2004). The impact of a "Promotora" on increasing routine chronic disease prevention among women aged 40 and older at the U.S.-Mexico border. *Health Education & Behavior, 31*(4), 185–285.

Ingram, H., Laney, N. K., & Gillilan, D. M. (1995). *Divided waters: Bridging the U.S.-Mexico Border.* Tucson, AZ: University of Arizona Press.

Ingram, M., Gallegos, G., & Elenes, J. (2005). Diabetes is a community issue: The critical elements of a successful outreach and education model on the U.S.-Mexico border. *Preventing Chronic Disease, 2*(1), A15.

Institute of Medicine. (2001). *Crossing the quality chasm: A new health system for the 21st century.* Washington, DC: National Academies Press.

Institute of Medicine. (2012). *How far have we come in reducing health disparities?: Progress since 2000: Workshop summary.* Washington, DC: The National Academies Press.

Jepson, R. G., Harris, F. M., Platt, S., & Tannahill, C. (2010). The effectiveness of interventions to change six health behaviors: A review of reviews. *BMC Public Health, 10*, 538. doi:10.1186/1471-2458-10-538.

Kluckhohn, C. (1951). The study of culture. In D. Lerner & H. D. Lasswell (Eds.), *The policy sciences* (pp. 86–101). Stanford: Stanford University Press.

Koh, H. K., Oppenheimer, S. C., Massin-Short, S. B., Emmons, K. M., Geller, A. C., & Viswanath, K. (2010). Translating research evidence into practice to reduce health disparities: A social determinants approach. *American Journal of Public Health, 100*, 572–580.

Kozel, C. T., Hubbell, A. P., Dearing, J. W., Kane, W. M., et al. (2006). Exploring agenda-setting for Healthy Border 2010: Research directions and methods. *Californian Journal of Health Promotion, 4*(1), 141–161.

Krieger, N. (1994). Epidemiology and the web of causation: Has anyone seen the spider? *Social Science and Medicine, 39*(7), 887–903.

Kumanyika, S. (2012). Health disparities research in global perspective: New insights and new directions. *Annual Review of Public Health, 33*, 1–5.

Lara, J. (1998). Health outreach programs in the colonias of the U.S.-Mexico border. In J. G. Power & T. Byrd (Eds.), *U.S.-Mexico border health: Issues for regional and migrant populations* (pp. 208–214). Thousand Oaks, CA: Sage.

Link, B. G. & Phelan, J. (1995). Social conditions as fundamental causes of disease. *Journal of Health and Social Behavior, 36*(Special Issue), 80–94.

Lobato, M. N. in collaboration with Work Group members (2001). Preventing and controlling tuberculosis along the U.S.-Mexico border. MMWR January 19, 2001/50(RR1); 1–2.

Mabry, P. L., Olster, D. H., Morgan, G. D., & Abrams, D. B. (2008). Interdisciplinarity and systems science to improve population health. *American Journal of Preventive Medicine, 35*(2 Suppl), S211–S224.

Marquez, R. R., & Romo, H. D. (Eds.). (2008). *Transformations of La Familia on the U.S.-Mexico border*. Notre Dame, IN: University of Notre Dame Press.

Martinez, O. J. (1994). *Border people. Life and society in the U.S.-Mexico borderlands*. Tucson: University of Arizona Press.

McLeroy, K. R., Bibeau, D., Steckler, A., & Glanz, K. (1988). An ecological perspective on health promotion programs. *Health Education Quarterly, 15*(4), 351–377.

Milardo, R. M. (1988). Families and social networks: An overview of theory and methodology. In R. M. Milardo (Ed.), *Families and social networks* (pp. 13–47). Thousand Oaks, CA: Sage.

Moyer, L. B., Brouwer, K. C., Brodine, S. K., Ramos, R., Lozada, R., Firestone Cruz, M., et al. (2008). Barriers and missed opportunities to HIV testing among injection users in two Mexico-U.S. border cities. *Drug Alcohol Review, 27*(1), 39–45.

Murphy, S. (1998). A mile away and a world apart: The impact of interdependent and independent views of the self on U.S.-Mexican communications. In J. G. Power & T. Byrd (Eds.), *US-Mexico border health: Issues for regional and migrant populations* (pp. 3–23). Thousand Oaks, CA: Sage.

National Immigration Forum (2012). The "Border Bubble": A look at spending on U.S. Borders. November, 2012. http://www.ruralhomes.org/storage/documents/colonias_infosheet.pdf

Organista, K. C., Carrillo, H., & Ayala, G. (2004). HIV prevention with Mexican migrants: Review, critique, and recommendations. *JAIDS Journal of Acquired Immune Deficiency Syndromes, 37*, S227–S239.

Pan American Health Organization (PAHO). (2012). *United States-Mexico border area in Health in the Americas, 2012 edition, country volume* (pp. 698–720). El Paso, TX: Pan American Field Office.

Pastor, R. A., & Castaneda, J. G. (1988). *Limits to friendship. The United States and Mexico*. New York: Vintage Books.

Peach, J. (2012). The aging of the border population. In E. Lee & P. Ganster (Eds.), *The U.S.-Mexico border environment: Progress and challenges for sustainability* (Vol. 16, pp. 17–53)., SCERP Monograph Series San Diego, CA: San Diego State University Press.

Ramiriz, A. G., McAlister, A., Gallion, K. J., & Villarreal, R. (1995). Targeting Hispanic populations: Future research and prevention strategies. *Environmental Health Perspectives, 103*, 287–290.

Ramiriz, A., Thompson, J. A., & Vela, L. (Eds.). (2013). *The South Texas health status review: A health disparities roadmap*. San Antonio: Institute for Health Promotion Research, U.T. Health Science Center.

Rashid, J. R., Spengler, R. F., Wagner, R. M., Melanson, C., Skillen, E. L., Mays, R. A., et al. (2009). Eliminating health disparities through transdisciplinary research, cross-agency collaboration, and public participation. *American Journal of Public Health, 99*(11), 1955–1961.

Resnicow, K., & Braithwaite, R. (2001). Cultural sensitivity in public health. In R. Braithwaite & S. Taylor (Eds.), *Health issues in the black community* (2nd ed.). San Francisco, CA: Jossey-Bass.

Rodriquez-Saldana, J. (2005). Challenges and opportunities in border health. *Preventing Chronic Disease, 2*(1), A03.

Ruark, E. & Martin, J. (2009). The sinking lifeboat: Uncontrolled immigration and the U.S. health care system in 2009. Federation for American Immigration Reform. Updated version of original 2004 report. Washington, DC.

Ruiz-Beltran, M., & Kamau, J. K. (2001). The socio-economic and cultural impediments to well-being along the U.S.-Mexico border. *Journal of Community Health, 26*(2), 123–132.

Rust, G., & Cooper, L. A. (2007). How can practice-based research contribute to the elimination of health disparities? *Journal of the American Board of Family Medicine, 20*(2), 105–114.

Schnittker, J., & McLeod, J. D. (2005). The social psychology of health disparities. *Annual Review of Sociology, 31*, 75–103.

Sellis, J. F., Owen, N., & Fisher, E. B. (2008). Ecological models of health behavior. In K. Glanz, B. K. Rimer, & K. Viswanath (Eds.), *Health behavior and health education: Theory, research, and practice* (pp. 465–485). San Francisco, CA: Jossey-Bass.

Sherif, M., Harvey, O. J., White, B. J., Hood, W. R., & Sherif, C. W. (1961). *Intergroup conflict and cooperation: The robbers cave experiment*. Norman, Oklahoma: Institute of Group Relations, University of Oklahoma.

Smedley, B. D., Stith, A. Y., & Nelson, A. R. (Eds.). (2003). *Unequal treatment: Confronting racial and ethnic disparities in health care*. Washington, DC: Institute of Medicine, The National Academies Press.

Smith, G. & Malkin, E. (1997). The border. Business week, May 12. Accessed at http://www.businessweek.com/1997/19/635261.htm

Southwest Center for Environmental Research and Policy (SCERP) (2012). U.S.-Mexican border region and border 2012 program: Environmental indicators.

Steinfelt, V. E. (2005). The border health strategic initiative from a community perspective. Preventing chronic disease, http://www.cdc.gov/pcd/issues/2005/jan/04_0077.htm

Syme, S. L. (2004). Social determinants of health: The community as an empowered partner. *Preventing Chronic Disease, 1*(1), 1–5.

Terrazas, A. (2010). Mexican immigrants in the United States. Migration information source, February, 2010. Accessed source @migrationpolicy.org. Accessed at http://www.immigrationinformation.org/usfocus/display.cfm?ID=767

Thomas, S. B., Fine, M. J., & Ibrahim, S. A. (2004). Health disparities: The importance of culture and health communication. *American Journal of Public Health, 94*(12), 2050.

U.S. Department of Environmental Protection Agency (2012). Clean energy and climate change-U.S.-Mexico Border. Accessed www.epa.gov/region9/climatechange/border.html

U.S. Department of Health and Human Services. (2005). *Eliminating health disparities: Measurement and data needs*. Washington, DC: National Academies Press.

U.S. Department of Health and Human Services (2011). National healthcare disparities report 2011. AHRQ Publication No. 12-006, Rockville, MD.

U.S. Department of Health and Human Services (2013). National healthcare disparities report 2012. AHRQ Publication No. 13-003, Rockville, MD.

U.S. Department of State (2012). Mexico. Accessed http://m.state.gov/md35749.htm

U.S. Department of Transportation (DOT) (2012). Bureau of transportation statistics, U.S.-Mexico border crossing data. Accessed from http://www.bts.gov/programs/international/border_crossing_entry_data/us_mexico/

U.S. Public Law 106-525. Minority health and health disparities research and education Act of 2000. 106th congress 2nd session, November 22, 2000.

U.S.-Mexico Border Health Commission (2003). Healthy border 2010: An agenda for improving health on the United States-Mexico border. A conference held at New Mexico State University, Las Cruces, October 2-4, 2003.

U.S.-Mexico Border Health Commission. (2010a). *Border Lives: Health status in the United States-Mexico Border Region*. El Paso, TX: U.S.-Mexico Border Health Commission.

U.S.-Mexico Border Health Commission (2010b). Health disparities and the U.S.-Mexico border: Challenges and opportunities. A White paper, October 25. El Paso, TX.

Valenzuela, G. E. (1992). The floating population of the border. In J. R. Weeks & R. Ham-Chande (Eds.), *Demographic dynamics of the U.S.-Mexico border* (pp. 187–200). El Paso, TX: Texas Western Press.

Waitzkin, H., Getrich, C., Heying, S., Pamar, A., Willging, C., Yager, J., et al. (2011). Promotoras as mental health practitioners in primary care: A multi-method study of an intervention to address contextual sources of depression. *Journal of Community Health, 36*(2), 316–331.

Webb, M. S., Rodriguez-Esquivel, D., & Baker, E. A. (2010). Smoking cessation interventions among Hispanics in the United States: A systematic review and mini meta-analysis. *American Journal of Health Promotion, 25*(2), 109–118.

Wilber, K. (1981). *No boundary*. Boston, MA: New Science Library.

Wilkinson, R. G. (1996). *Unhealthy societies: The afflictions of inequality* (pp. 1–9 and 12–21). New York: Routledge.

Williams, R. A. (2011). Historical perspectives of healthcare disparities. In R. A. Williams (Ed.), *Healthcare disparities at the crossroads with healthcare reform* (pp. 7–21). New York: Springer.

Woolf, S. H., Johnson, R. E., Fryer, G. E., Rust, G., & Satcher, D. (2004). The health impact of resolving racial disparities: An analysis of U.S. mortality data. *American Journal of Public Health, 94*(12), 2078–2080.

Chapter 2
Understanding Health Disparities

2.1 Introduction

Along with a broader definition of health, our view of disease causation and predisease pathways has also broadened as it has become clear that health risks are created and maintained by social systems and that the magnitude of those risks are largely a function of socioeconomic and psychosocial disparities (Halfon and Hochstein 2002). Therefore, our efforts to reduce health disparities can no longer be confined to only providing better access and more resources to meet the needs of the underserved. We must address the underlying social factors that determine health disparities. Too much emphasis is placed on individual lifestyle choices. We tend to forget that lifestyles are largely determined by social, economic, and environmental determinants.

Disparities in health outcomes and in the factors contributing to them are present early in life and are expressed and compounded by experiences during a person's lifetime. Risk factors are part of a person's biological make-up, embedded in the disparities of a family or community, and maintained by social, cultural, and economic forces in a given society.

There are multiple road maps to health, but one pathway that has emerged most strongly is the association between people's material circumstances or relative income, and health. What is important is how the level of material prosperity places an individual in relation to others. Projects designed to improve people's jobs and education do not change the sum total of disadvantage (Wilkinson 1999). There are a host of factors embedded in the phenomenon of poverty so there is no single explanation for socioeconomic differences in health. The cumulative effects of the multiple hardships of material disadvantage are disproportionate and synergistic, rather than additive. Therefore, piecemeal strategies for improving health among lower socioeconomic groups are not usually effective (Dutton and Levine 1989).

A 2010 Gallop survey of 200,000 Americans across incomes documents the severity of health disparities between low and high income Americans. Those making less than $24,000 per year suffer from poorer emotional and physical

J. G. Bruhn, *Culture and Health Disparities*, SpringerBriefs in Public Health,
DOI: 10.1007/978-3-319-06462-8_2, © The Author(s) 2014

health, have poorer health habits, and have significantly less access to medical care (Mendes 2010). Low-income Americans are in a negative health feedback cycle—they have poorer health habits and high levels of physical illness, less access to preventive care and treatment, and live with heightened emotional negativity about breaking the cycle. Health disparities seem to be becoming more embedded at a time when more people are facing financial hardships. One-third of low-income Americans are uninsured and more than that say that there have been times when they didn't have enough money for healthcare (Mendes 2010).

Poor health is interwoven with the position of the poor in the social structure and larger culture of our society. The different ways to measure socioeconomic status be they income, education or occupation, yield a roughly similar picture of health inequities with common social consequences such as alienation. Inequalities in both health and economic status have persisted over decades and appear to be increasing. While most American men and women experience increasing longevity, less advantaged groups experience levels of longevity comparable to men and women in developing countries. Inequalities in health in the United States occur among both sexes and all ages, and for many people the detrimental effects of poverty on health begin in early life and worsen as they live to old age. The overlap between poverty and minority status creates a double jeopardy that deprives the poor of ever experiencing good health.

It is an established fact in rich societies the poor have shorter lives and suffer more from almost every social problem. Wilkinson and Pickett (2009) found one common factor that links the healthiest and happiest societies, the degree of equality among their members. Almost every current social problem—poor health, violence, lack of community life, teen pregnancy and mental illness—is more likely to occur in a less-equal society. That is why, according to Wilkinson and Pickett, America, the richest nation on earth, has per capita shorter life spans, more mental illness, more obesity, and more people in prison than any other developed nation. The social links between health and inequality draw attention to the fact that social, rather than material, factors are now the limiting component in the quality of life in developed societies (Wilkinson 1996).

In more egalitarian societies and parts of societies where there are smaller differences in income between rich and poor, the average health standards of the population are better and there is greater longevity. Egalitarian societies are also more socially cohesive (Wilkinson 1996). Many of the socioeconomic determinants of health have their effects through psychosocial pathways. There is strong evidence that the pathway is from income distribution through social relationships to health. In societies where income differences are larger, social environment is less supportive, there is a greater proportion of people who feel that they cannot trust others, and there is a higher rate of aggression toward other people and their property. James (1995) found evidence that income inequality and poverty increases stress on family life leading to more domestic violence and to more children growing up to become violent adults. The quality of people's social relationships has a powerful influence on their health.

Marmot (2004) views social inequities as the major causes of ill-health. He calls this "the status syndrome." The status syndrome is not simply one of income or lifestyle differences; it is the psychological experience of inequality that has a profound influence on health. Marmot believes if we can understand social inequalities, we can mitigate their effects.

Why should our society care about income inequality? Kawachi and Kennedy (1997) pointed out that income inequality has spillover effects on the quality of life of a society, for example, the middle class flight from poor neighborhoods results in the progressive deterioration of public education. Those who are economically disadvantaged are also likely to be temporarily or permanently unemployed leading to their low productivity and contributing to the slower economic growth of the communities where they live. Income inequality threatens the functioning of democracy when the poor express low levels of trust in others, especially trust in their government. Therefore, it is not surprising that the poor are underrepresented among voters in our country. Wide income disparities tend to coexist with underinvestment in human capital measured by high school dropout rates, reduced public spending on education, and lower literacy rates. Finally, wide income disparities result in frustration, stress, and family disruption, which in turn, increase rates of violence, crime, and homicide in society as a whole (Wilkinson 1996).

2.2 Health Disparities: Definitions and Perspectives

According to the Centers for Disease Control and Prevention (CDC) health disparities are preventable differences in the burden of disease, injury, violence, or opportunities to achieve optimal health that are experienced by socially disadvantaged populations (CDC 2005, 2008). Health disparities are inequities that are directly related to the historical and current unequal distribution of social, political, economic, and environmental resources (U.S. Department of Health and Human Services 2010/2020).

The Institute of Medicine (2000) has defined disparities as differences in treatment provided to members of different groups that are not justified by the underlying health conditions or treatment preferences of patients (Smedley et al. 2003).

Disparities fall along a continuum from being minimally unjust to overt discrimination. At what point along the continuum differences become disparities is subjective, but the magnitude of the injustice and disparity is generally thought to be proportional to how much control individuals and groups have over the cause(s) of the differences (Herbert et al. 2008).

There is little consensus on what constitutes a disparity because disparities are not discrete or always easily observed and therefore their size or extent is unknown and not easily measureable. Therefore, one of the ways to reduce disparities is to strive for equity in health and healthcare services for all groups (U.S. Dept. of HHS 2011).

Health inequities have been growing in the U.S. and creating gaps in the distribution of illness, healthcare, and longevity. In public health these inequities are viewed as unnecessary, avoidable, and are considered unjust (Satcher 2010). They are maintained over time beyond the control of individuals (Hofrichter 2010).

Inequities are embedded in the history and culture of societies. They are matrixed in the structure of social, economic, and political institutions, and are expressed in various forms of social exclusion and exploitation. Changes in health policy alone have not and cannot solve the problem of health inequalities (Adler et al. 1993).

There are many groups of people in the U.S. who, for reasons of disability, color, income, sexual orientation and language, are disconnected from social institutions, and therefore are unable to access resources to obtain the basic necessities of life including health and child care, transportation, housing, and education. House and Williams (2000) explain, "....over the life course individuals first acquire varying levels and types of education, which in turn help them enter various types of occupations, which then yield income, which finally enables them to accumulate assets or wealth. Each subsequent factor in this chain of events is affected by prior variables." p. 83. Because inequalities are interconnected through their related causes and effects, they can be framed and understood through a social systems perspective (Robert and House 2000).

2.3 The Development of Health Disparities

2.3.1 The Life Course Model

The life course model of health provides a framework for understanding how children's health and environmental exposures are connected to the development of disorders, disability, and death among adults (Halfon and Hochstein 2002). This model proposes that health disparities exist across the life span but that childhood is a critical period in their development. Unique interactions occur at each stage of development which can generate or create risks for subsequent layers of disparities. Longitudinal data confirm that health disparities change as individuals move through the life course (Pavalko and Caputo 2013). Obesity in early childhood is an example of how being overweight at an early age increases the risk in adulthood of mortality and morbidity from coronary heart disease, colorectal cancer, and arthritis (Forrest and Riley 2004). The life course model also provides insights into adaptive mechanisms or social resiliency factors such as social support used to maximize health-enhancing capacities at various points in life (Pearlin et al. 2005). A major focus of the life course perspective has been to understand how early-life experiences shape adult health, particularly adult chronic disease and its risk factors and consequences (Braveman and Barclay 2009).

The development of health disparities in the U.S.-Mexico border region begins with birth and the high infant mortality rates per 1,000 live births for Mexico and the U.S. border (Fig. 2.1) (Woolf and Braveman 2011). These high rates are due to poor pre-natal services and utilization, low rates of immunization, and the adverse physical environment children are exposed to. Indeed, as many as 40 % of children who survive infancy grow up in the circumstances of poverty in a border state (Fig. 2.2). If the child survives and enters school the drop-out rate for Latino teens aged 16–19 years living in the Southwest is 15 % compared to non-Latinos (5 %)

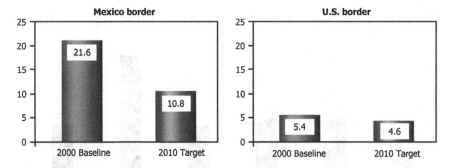

Fig. 2.1 Infant mortality. *Source* United States: National Center for Health Statistics, CDC. Mexico: INEGI/SSA, 2000

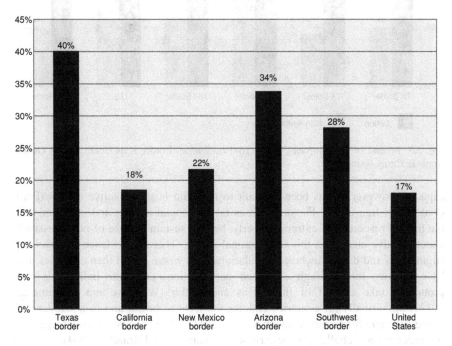

Fig. 2.2 Percent of children in poverty, 2000. *Source* Border Kids Count Pocket Guide, Annie E. Casey Foundation

(see Fig. 2.3). Teenage births on the border are higher (17 %) than for the U.S. as a whole (12 %). Childhood obesity is at epidemic proportions with 22 % of 4th graders being obese and 39 % being overweight (U.S.-Mexico Border Health Commission 2010; LaFe Policy and Advocacy Center 2006).

Health and the general quality of life along the U.S.-Mexico border, especially in the colonias, has been a victim to systemic social and economic injustices (Lusk et al. 2012). Isolated efforts have been made primarily at local levels to advance health promotion and disease prevention, develop leaders, and build community

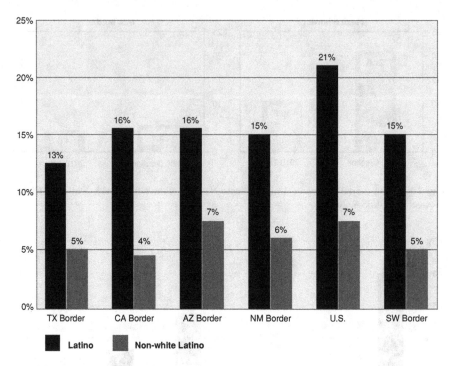

Fig. 2.3 Percent of HS Dropouts, teens (16–19). *Source* Border Kids Count Pocket Guide, Annie E. Casey Foundation

capacity, however, it has been difficult to maintain lasting positive effects (Ford et al. 1998; Iton 2010). Factors such as racism, social neglect and isolation, and the limited resources of extreme poverty, help to sustain a sense of powerlessness about positive change in this international region. There is evidence that racially stigmatized and disenfranchised populations have worse health than countries that have policies that through enhanced participation, empower individuals and groups to take control of their lives and health (Williams and Mohammed 2013a, b). Virtually all countries endorse the right to health and to a standard of living adequate for health (Braveman et al. 2011).[1] The persistence and deepening of border poverty challenges these rights (Mondragon and Brandon 2004).

2.4 Causes of Border Health Disparities

Iton (2010) points out that wealth is the strongest determinant of health in the United States and many developed countries. It is the means by which individuals access a variety of social and health benefits. Although health is consistently worse

---

[1] There are different definitions of health disparities or inequalities. International definitions focus on socioeconomic differences, while in the U.S. health disparities often refer to racial or ethnic differences. For a discussion of definitions see Braveman et al. (2011).

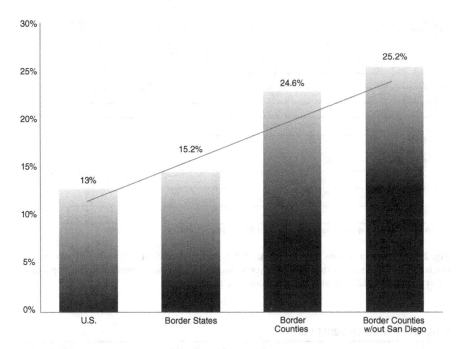

Fig. 2.4 Percent Living below poverty level in the U.S. and border region. *Data source* U.S. Census Bureau, ACS, 2008

for individuals with few resources, the degree of health disparities in the U.S. varies by race/ethnicity, income, time and geographic location (Adler and Rehkopf 2008).

The single most substantial source of health disparities in the U.S. and U.S.-Mexico border is poverty (Pettit and Nienhaus 2010) (see Fig. 2.4). Figure 2.5 shows a 52-year perspective of poverty in the U.S. from 1959 to 2011. The poverty rate in the U.S. in 2011 was 15 % or 46.2 million individuals, the highest rate since 1993. This is one indicator that the U.S. health status is slipping. Other developed countries have lower child poverty rates and maintain a stronger safety net to help disadvantaged families maintain their health (Woolf and Braveman 2011).

Table 2.1 shows the breakdown of poverty in the U.S. for the general population, for Latinos, and for children. Within the Latino community people living in poverty reached record numbers in 2011; more than 13 million individuals.

Nearly 15 % of Latino households experienced food insecurity, the rate for children under 18 being 34.5 % (see Table 2.2).[2]

---

[2] Income levels of the communities on the U.S. side are below the U.S. national average, whereas income levels of communities on the Mexican side are above the Mexican national average. The situation is reflected in the poverty rates, which tend to be higher than the national average on the U.S. side and lower than the national average on the Mexican side. In other words, the income gap and poverty rate differences in the border region are smaller than the differences between those same measures for the two countries as a whole. See Anderson and Gerber (2008). Also, Centers for Disease Control and Prevention (2005). Also, U.S. Dept. HHS (2011).

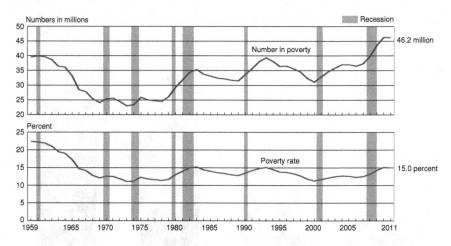

Fig. 2.5 Number in poverty & poverty rate: 1959–2011, United States. *Note* The data points are placed at the midpoints of the respective years. *Source* U.S. Census Bureau, Current Population Survey. 1990 to 2012 Annual Social and Economic Supplements

Table 2.1 U.S. Poverty, 2011 Data

	General population (%)	Latinos (%)
Individuals	15.0	25.3
Children under 18	21.9	34.1
Children under 5	25.1	36.0

Source U.S. Census Bureau
Household Food Security in the United States in 2011. U.S. Department of Agriculture, Economic Research Service, September 2012

Table 2.2 Food insecurity, 2011

	U.S. general population	U.S. Latinos
Households	14.9 %	26.2 %
	17.9 million	3.8 million
Individuals	16.4 %	28.3 %
	50.1 million	13.8 million
Children under 18	22.4 %	34.5 %
	16.7 million	5.5 million

Source USDA Economic Research Service
Statistical Supplement to Household Food Security in the United States in 2011. U.S. Department of Agriculture, Economic Research Service, September 2012

Three of the ten poorest counties in the U.S. are located in the border region. Twenty-one of the counties on the border have been designated as economically distressed areas.

2.5 Colonias

The colonias are one of the border regions' largest pockets of poverty. Mexican Americans living in colonias are one of the most disadvantaged, hard to reach minority groups in the U.S. (Mier et al. 2008). A colonias is a rural shanty town or colony characterized by poor housing, inadequate physical structure, and a weak social infrastructure. Colonias are a form of self-help housing settlement. In the 1990s colonias became a common name for the slums that developed on both sides of the U.S.-Mexico border. While colonias have existed along the border for decades, the signing of the North Atlantic Free Trade Agreement (NAFTA) in 1994 has significantly increased the number of people living in colonias due, in part, to the low-paying jobs in maquiladoras.

There is no formal census of colonia residents as lots are acquired informally, no subdivisions are recorded, and there are no community development offices. Estimates are that approximately half a million people lived in 2,000 colonias in Texas in 2007. Texas has the largest concentration of people living in colonias on the U.S. side of the border. New Mexico has the second largest, followed by Arizona and California. Over 50 % of colonias have fewer than 2,000 residents; only seven colonias exceed 10,000 population. Overall, these communities lack infrastructure (paved roads, water and sewer systems, and electricity), have high levels of poverty, high unemployment, limited health care and educational opportunities, and a disproportionate number of Hispanics. Colonias are often defined by what they lack. There is a persistence of physical infrastructure deficiencies. The civic infrastructure lacks consistent, strong leaders. Colonias continue to attract poor people. There are insufficient funds at all levels to address basic needs (Esparza and Donelson 2008).

Despite being categorized, colonias vary within the border region from small clusters of homes near agricultural employment opportunities to established communities whose residents commute to nearby urban centers (Table 2.3). Also, colonias have varied histories; some have been in existence since the 19th century while others have emerged in the last 50 years.

Despite their growth in the 1950s colonias have remained unnoticed until 1990 when a federal definition of colonias was created.[3] In the U.S. border counties, 25–30 % of the population is uninsured. The average yearly income is $14,500. Educational attainment is lower when compared to the rest of the U.S. and unemployment is 250–300 % higher than that of the rest of the U.S. Estimates are that 85 % of colonia residents are U.S. citizens.

Hispanic residents along the border experience poverty at more than twice the U.S. rate. Most colonias residents work in nearby cities, primarily in low-wage

---

[3] In 1990 the Cranston-Gonzalez National Affordable Housing Act (NAHA) created a federal definition for colonias. Under NAHA a colonia is an "identifiable community" in Arizona, California, New Mexico, or Texas within 150 miles of the U.S.-Mexico border, lacking decent water and sewage systems and decent housing and in existence as a colonia before November 28, 1989.

Table 2.3 U.S. border Colonias

	Rural border colonias	Border colonias	United States
Population	1,650,448	5,586,664	301,461,533
Hispanic population (%)	52.0	61.8	15.1
Poverty rate (%)	20.7	23.8	13.5
Population living in small town/rural (%)	100	29.8	21.2
Homeownership (%)	72.7	67.7	66.9

Source Border Colonias Housing Assistance Council (*HAC*) Tabulations of the American Community Survey 2005–2009 Five Year Estimates

service jobs and in manufacturing and food processing activities. The colonias are also home for many migrant farmworkers, but they are only a small part of the population.

Although there have been significant economic changes due to international trade agreements, major problems associated with general poverty continue to exist. Without sustained federal, state and local government and private funding for health programs, infrastructure and education, the border population will continue to lag behind the rest of the U.S. (U.S.-Mexico Border Commission 2010; Rodriguez-Saldana 2005).

2.6 The Poor and Homeless: Embedded Disparities

Poverty lingers in the U.S. as it does in other parts of the world. The usual reasons for the persistence of poverty are the lack of education and skills, lack of the opportunity to change one's social class, lack of social, human and economic capital, discrimination, and imperialism.

Other reasons why poverty lingers is that it has deep generational roots, pessimistic attitudes, and the loss of hope that things will change.

There are connections between poverty and homelessness. Not all poor are homeless, but all homeless are poor. The homeless are drawn from a pool of the extremely poor (Auletta 1999; Rossi 1989). Poverty and homelessness have been identified as two of several indicators of the social health of the U.S. The Fordham Institute for Innovation in Social Policy has studied indicators of the social health of America and published trends in these indicators each year since 1987, to increase public awareness of social conditions (Miringhoff and Miringhoff 1999). Like economic indexes, the Index of Social Health uses key social indicators that assess the quality of life such as child abuse, suicide, drug abuse, health care, and core socioeconomic indicators that measure well-being, including average income, poverty, and inequities.

Poverty and homelessness are not one problem, but many; they are not a condition, but the result of a process; the societal resources needed to assist them are chronically inadequate because we only deal with the most visible part of disparities. One of the limitations in increasing our understanding of the process of becoming poor and homeless is our tendency to stereotype so that the poor and homeless are viewed as homogeneous.

We usually hear that people "fall" into poverty and once fallen, they cannot "climb" out of it. The "fall" is usually attributed to faults of the social structure or to individual shortcomings or failures. Cotter (2002) suggests that poverty is a multilevel problem. Poverty is a process of disconnectedness that involves individuals and families facing an accumulation of broken or breaking social connections to social institutions. Disconnectedness takes many forms, including joblessness, the inability to meet financial obligations and making severe and sudden changes in one's lifestyle. The rapidity of the progression into poverty is variable depending on individual and familial circumstances and the available alternatives (Trickett and Beehler 2013). Nevertheless, disconnecting from an acceptable lifestyle to a stigmatized one is an experience of profound loss.

Similarly, homelessness is a process of disconnectedness. The homeless are not only poor but they have no place to live—they carry their identity with them. One of the key predictors of being poor and homeless is a family history of poverty and homelessness; these problems are generational and cyclical. Most youth who are homeless have experienced broken, rejecting, hateful, and oftentimes violent relationships in their families.

2.7   Health-Related Quality of Life in Colonias

Social and health disparities are prominent among Mexican-Americans who live along the border (Anderson and Gerber 2008; Barr 2008). Studies have shown that health-related quality of life is associated with poverty, low levels of education, being Hispanic or black, older age, female gender, disability, inability to work, unemployment, lifestyle behaviors, and chronic disease (Mier et al. 2008). Few studies have examined the health profile of Mexican-American adults living in colonias. One study obtained a high response rate (87 %) among adults 18 years and over living in three separate colonias in Texas. These researchers used trained interviewers who conducted face-to-face interviews in Spanish (Mier et al. 2008). Results showed that participants reported worse physical health compared to the U.S. population norm and Hispanic norm. Despite adverse living conditions in the colonias participants reported a level of mental health similar to the U.S. and Hispanic norms. Living in the colonias for ten years or more and a low level of education predicted poor physical and mental health. Poor mental health was associated with the perception that accessing healthcare services was problematic for colonias residents. Results from this study suggest that colonias residents, especially residents of ten years or more may have adapted to the limitations of their environment and their ability to access healthcare. In other words, colonias residents' expectations regarding healthcare are realistic given their circumstances of living in extreme poverty.

2.8 Pathways to Poverty

There is a large body of literature to support the theory that family poverty adversely affects children's health through increased neonatal and post-neonatal mortality rates, lower intellectual capabilities, lower academic achievement, greater risk of injuries resulting from accidents or physical abuse/neglect, higher risk for asthma, and lower developmental scores on a range of tests at multiple ages (Weitzman 2007; Aber et al. 1997). Children who experience poverty during their preschool and early school years have lower rates of school completion than children and adolescents who experience poverty in later years (Brooks-Gunn and Duncan 1997; Leventhal and Brooks-Gunn 2000). Yet, we know little about the pathways by which poverty exerts its negative influence. Some models have been suggested (social systems; ecological) but there is no consensus on how poverty should be operationalized so that proposed models can be refined and tested (Aber et al. 1997).

Researchers emphasize that studies of socioeconomic inequalities should begin early in the life course. Poverty occurring early in childhood may cause developmental damage that affects individuals and families for a lifetime. Poverty is a dynamic variable; therefore data need to be gathered longitudinally to capture the effects of poverty at various life stages. Research methodology needs to be comprehensive yet, in depth enough to measure time-dependent variables.

2.9 Conceptualization of a Social Systems Approach to Understanding Health Disparities

Our knowledge of pathways or mechanisms of disparities has been limited because the focus has been on static variables rather than on process variables; the former can be quantified and measured while process variables are subjective, broad and interrelated. Indeed, pathways research requires a longitudinal research methodology of repeated assessments of variables over time. Process variables are usually interrelated with other process variables as well as with static ones. The interconnectedness of process variables is why disparities do not have identified beginning and ending points; they are a web of dynamic connections in a continually changing system.

Figure 2.6 presents a suggested social systems approach to understanding health disparities. A social systems approach is especially relevant to poverty because it is in constant flux and its causes and consequences exist at all levels of a social system. Figure 2.6 illustrates the interrelationships between the United States and Mexico at many levels in both cultures. The figure also illustrates the different types of data needed to focus on poverty and its corollaries of marginalization and homelessness. While the figure is presented as if the intervention process is linear it is in fact cyclical, relational and tied to the life cycle of individuals, neighborhoods and communities.

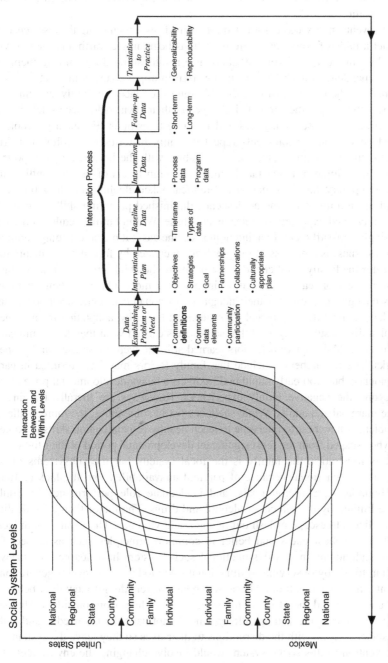

Fig. 2.6 A social systems approach to understanding health disparities

Whitbeck and Hoyt (1999), in a study of 602 runaways and homeless adolescents, identified variables that put youth at risk for poverty, homelessness, and marginalization.

A life events matrix was constructed for each adolescent enabling the researchers to construct a table of consecutive life transitions beginning at birth and ending with the adolescent's current living situation. The results showed a recurring theme or early independence for children resulting from multiple changes in caretakers and in residence. The more transitions the children experienced in family structure and residence, the earlier they initiated change on their own. Adolescents left homes characterized by loose family ties and multiple transitions. Frequently, problems spanned generations. Adolescents repeated family histories of alcohol and drug problems, mental health problems, and troubles with the law. The family portrait was one of multiple troubled family members, high levels of family conflict, and fragile, temporary family situations. Parent/caretaker alcohol and drug problems resulted in discomfort for the adolescents, diminished parenting skills of caretakers, and increased exposure to violence and abuse. Within families children became increasingly self-sufficient. Leaving home became easy; it meant escaping conflict.

Homelessness is a process of marginalization created by forced early maturation. The greater the family conflict and abuse the more the child separates from the family. The process of leaving separates him/her even more. Once on their own their options change; they transfer their allegiance to nonadults. Same aged social networks have critical developmental consequences; to get by, adaptation involves new survival skills. Results suggested that adolescents carried what they knew into early independence. Maladaptive behaviors learned at home were those used in their new networks. The researchers conclude that family factors may have resulted in early independence, but "too-early adulthood" extracts a heavy developmental price above and beyond the negative family experiences. Runaways are literally learning to become marginalized adults. While shelters exist in some cities, the more challenging problem is how best to intervene to teach healthy resocialization skills to adolescents who escaped from the most significant developmental period of their lives.

In this illustration the family is the focal system, but the subsystems of the family are dysfunctional because of parental unavailability and the lack of functional boundaries, common goals, and inadequate role performance by adults who are limited by the effects of alcohol and drugs. The major theme for dealing with conflict is to escape or lash out in anger and violence. The focal system lacks integrity and cohesiveness and belief in common principles such as respect for persons. Individuals in this dysfunctional social system have learned to survive, not adapt, to life by observing dysfunctional role models over several generations. Input into this system is limited because the key players do not view their behavior as dysfunctional and therefore do not see a need for help from outsiders. The output of the system is the young children who do not have the knowledge and skills or assistance to cope with the disruptions to their lives so they leave the system.

Intervention in this social system would involve changing the environment for the runaways, exposing them to healthy adults and peers, through teaching and mentoring helping them to see and practice healthy alternatives to their behavior.

This process will take resources, time, patience, reinforcement, and monitoring to keep the runaway interested, motivated, and supported so the appeal of a life of self-sufficiency does not draw them back to the street.

2.10 Summary

There is substantial literature on the relationship between health disparities, especially poverty, on the development of children, in particular the negative effects that follow children throughout their life cycle. The problem with existing research findings is that poverty and other disparities researchers do not gather longitudinal data so we know little about when and how health disparities interfere negatively with child development. Therefore, we do not understand how poverty is expressed as individuals and groups move through their life cycles. We have suggested that a social systems approach to health disparities will yield insights into how and when interventions can help to alter the momentum of poverty and its negative effects.

References

Aber, J. L., Bennett, N. G., Conley, D. C., & Li, J. (1997). The effects of poverty on child health and development. *Annual Review of Public Health, 18*, 463–483.

Adler, N. E., Boyce, W. T., Chesney, M. A., Folkman, S., & Syme, S. L. (1993). Socioeconomic inequalities in health: No easy solution. *Journal of the American Medical Association, 269*(24), 3140–3145.

Adler, N. E., & Rehkopf, D. H. (2008). U.S. disparities in health: Descriptions, causes, and mechanisms. *Annual Review of Public Health, 29*, 235–252.

Anderson, J. B. & Gerber, J. (2008). Fifty years of change on the U.S.-Mexico Border. Austin: University of Texas Press.

Auletta, K. (1999). *The underclass*. New York: The Overlook Press.

Barr, D. A. (2008). *Health disparities in the United States*. Baltimore: The Johns Hopkins Press.

Braveman, P., & Barclay, C. (2009). Health disparities beginning in childhood: A life-course perspective. *Pediatrics, 124*, S163–S175.

Braveman, P. A., Kumanyika, S., Fielding, J., LaVeist, T., Borrell, L. N., Manderscheid, R., et al. (2011). Health disparities and health equity: The issue is justice. *American Journal of Public Health, 101*(Supplement), 5149–5155.

Brooks-Gunn, J., & Duncan, G. J. (1997). The effects of poverty on children. *The Future of Children, 7*(2), 55–71.

Centers for Disease Control and Prevention (CDC). (2005). Racial/ethnic and socioeconomic disparities in multiple risk factors for heart disease and stroke. *United States 2003. Morbidity Mortality Weekly Reports, 54*(5), 113–117.

Centers for Disease Control and Prevention (CDC). (2008). Community Health and Program Services (CHAPS): Health disparities among racial/ethnic populations: Atlanta: Department of Health and Human Services.

Cotter, D. A. (2002). Poor people in poor places: Local opportunity structures and household poverty. *Rural Sociology, 67*(4), 534–555.

Dutton, D. B. & Levine, S. (1989). Socioeconomic status and health: Overview, methodological critique, and reformulation. In J. P. Bunker, D. S. Gomby, & B. H. Kehrer (Eds.), *Pathways to health: The role of social factors* (pp. 29–69). Menlo Park: The Henry J. Kaiser Family Foundation.

Esparza, A. X., & Donelson, A. J. (2008). *Colonias in Arizona and New Mexico: Border poverty and community.* Tucson: University of Arizona Press.

Ford, L. A., Barnes, M. D., Crabtree, R. D. & Fairbanks, J. (1998). Boundary spanners: Las promotoras in the borderlands. In J. G. Power & T. Byrd (Eds.), *U.S.-Mexico border health: Issues for regional and migrant populations* (pp. 141–164). Thousand Oaks: Sage.

Forrest, C. B., & Riley, A. W. (2004). Childhood origins of adult health: A basis for life-course health policy. *Health Affairs, 23*(5), 155–164.

Halfon, N., & Hochstein, M. (2002). Life course health development: An integrated framework for developing health policy and research. *Milbank Quarterly, 80*(3), 433–479.

Herbert, P. L., Sisk, J. E., & Howell, E. A. (2008). When does a difference become a disparity? Conceptualizing racial and ethnic disparities in health. *Health Affairs, 27*(2), 374–382.

Hofrichter, R. (2010). Tackling health inequities: A framework for public health practice. In R. Hofrichter & R. Bhatia (Eds.), *Tackling health inequities through public health practice: Theory to action* (2nd ed., pp. 3–56). New York: Oxford University Press.

House, J. S., & Williams, D. R. (2000). Understanding and reducing socioeconomic and racial/ethnic disparities in health. In B. D. Smedley & S. L. Syme (Eds.), *Promoting health: Intervention strategies from social and behavioral research* (pp. 81–124). Washington, DC: National Academy Press.

Institute of Medicine. (2000). *The future of the public's health in the 21st century.* Washington, DC: The National Academies Press.

Iton, A. (2010). Tackling the root causes of health disparities through community capacity building. In R. Hofrichter & R. Bhatia (Eds.), *Tackling health inequities through public health practice* (2nd ed.). New York: Oxford University Press.

James, O. (1995). *Juvenile violence in a winner-loser culture.* London: Free Association Books.

Kawachi, I., & Kennedy, B. P. (1997). Health and social cohesion: Why care about income inequality? *British Medical Journal, 314*, 1037–1040.

LaFe Policy & Advocacy Center (2006). CHC border health policy forum. The U.S.-Mexico border: Demographic, socio-economic, and health issues, Profile 1. San Antonio, Texas.

Leventhal, T., & Brooks-Gunn, J. (2000). The neighborhoods they live in: The effects of neighborhood residence on child and adolescent outcomes. *Psychological Bulletin, 126*(2), 309–337.

Lusk, M. W., Staudt, K. A., & Moya, E. (Eds.). (2012). *Social justice in the U.S.-Mexico border region.* New York: Springer.

Marmot, M. (2004). *The status syndrome: How social standing affects our health and longevity.* New York: Henry Holt & Co.

Mendes, E. (2010). In U.S., health disparities across incomes are wide-ranging. Gallup-healthways well-being index. http://www.gallup.com/

Mier, N., Ory, M. G., Zhan, D., Conkling, M., Sharkey, J. R., & Burdine, J. N. (2008). Health-related quality of life among Mexican Americans living in colonias at the Texas–Mexico border. *Social Science and Medicine, 66*, 1760–1771.

Miringhoff, M., & Miringhoff, M. (1999). *The social health of the nation: How America is really doing.* New York: Oxford University Press.

Mondragon, D., & Brandon, J. (2004). To address health disparities on the U.S.-Mexico Border—advances human rights. *Health and Human Rights: An International Journal, 8*(1), 179–195.

Pavalko, E. K., & Caputo, J. (2013). Social inequality and health access across the life course. *American Behavioral Scientist, 57*(8), 1040–1056.

Pearlin, L. I., Schleman, S., Fazio, E. M., & Meersman, S. C. (2005). Stress, health and the life course: Some conceptual perspectives. *Journal of Health and Social Behavior, 46*(2), 205–219.

Pettit, M. L. & Nienhaus, A. R. (2010). The current scope of health disparities in the U.S.: A review of literature. *The Health Educator, 42*(2), 47–55.

Robert, S. A., & House, J. S. (2000). Socioeconomic inequalities in health: Integrating individual-, community-, and societal-level theory and research. In G. L. Albrecht, R. Fitzpatrick, & S. C. Scrimshaw (Eds.), *Handbook of social studies in health and medicine* (pp. 115–135). Thousand Oaks: Sage.

Rossi, P. H. (1989). *Down and out in America: The origins of homelessness.* Chicago: University of Chicago.

Rodriguez-Saldana, J. (2005). Challenges and opportunities in border health. *Preventing Chronic Disease: Public Health Research, Practice, and Policy, 2*(1), 1–4.

Satcher, D. (2010). Include a social determinants of health approach to reduce health inequities. *Public Health Reports, 125*(Suppl. 4), 6–7.

Smedley, B. D., Stith, A. Y., & Nelson, A. R. (Eds.). (2003). *Unequal treatment: Confronting racial and ethnic disparities in health care.* Washington, DC: National Academies Press.

Trickett, E. J., & Beehler, S. (2013). The ecology of multilevel interventions to reduce social inequities in health. *American Behavioral Scientist, 57*(8), 1227–1246.

U.S. Department of Health and Human Services. (2010/2020). *Healthy people, 2010/2020: Understanding and improving health* (2nd ed.), Washington, DC.

U.S. Department of Health and Human Services. (2011). Centers for Disease Control. Health Disparities and Inequalities Report—United States, 2011. MMWR Supplement Vol. 60, January 14.

U.S. Mexico Border Commission. (2010). Health disparities and the U.S.-Mexico border: Challenges and opportunities. A white paper. October 25 2010.

Weitzman, M. (2007). Low income and its impact on psychosocial child development. In R. E. Tremblay, M. Boivin & R. DeV Peters (Eds.), *Encyclopedia on early childhood development* (2nd ed., pp. 1–8). Available at http://www.childencyclopedia.com/docuo nts/weitzmanANGxp.pdf

Whitbeck, L. B., & Hoyt, D. R. (1999). *Nowhere to grow: Homeless and runaway adolescents and their families.* New York: DeGruyter.

Wilkinson, R. G. (1996). *Unhealthy societies: The affliction of inequality.* New York: Routledge.

Wilkinson, R. G. (1999). Putting the picture together: Prosperity, redistribution, health and welfare. In M. Marmot & R. G Wilkinson (Eds.), *Social determinants of health* (pp. 256–274). New York: Oxford University Press.

Wilkinson, R., & Pickett, K. (2009). *The spirit level: Why greater equality makes societies stronger.* London: Bloomsbury Press.

Williams, D. R., & Mohammed, S. A. (2013a). Racism and health 11: A needed research agenda for effective interventions. *American Behavioral Scientist, 57*(8), 1200–1226.

Williams, D. R., & Mohammed, S. A. (2013b). Racism and health 1. Pathways and scientific evidence. *American Behavioral Scientist, 57*(8), 1152–1173.

Woolf, S. H., & Braveman, P. (2011). Where health disparities begin: The role of social and economic determinants—and why current policies may make matters worse. *Health Affairs, 30*(10), 1852–1859.

Chapter 3
A Critique of U.S.-Mexico Border Health Interventions

3.1 Introduction

The social and health needs and disparities of some twelve million Mexicans and Americans who reside along the U.S.-Mexico border continue to grow in complexity and severity despite numerous binational conferences, commissions, and agreements (U.S.-Mexico Border Health Commission 2003, 2010). Despite advocacy and information-sharing efforts, effective and sustained mechanisms for consensus-building on how best to intervene in various health problems, share "best practices," and replicate effective interventions, have not been widely developed and used. The understanding and resolution of the political, cultural, and social impediments to many common health issues remain substantial on both sides of the border (Homedes and Ugalde 2003, 2009; Ganster and Lorey 2008). Too much emphasis continues to be placed on "downstream" problems such as morbidity and mortality rates, the use and non-use of health services, and disease intervention with a curative focus. Kozel et al. (2006) propose a transformational process for redirecting the border health agenda "upstream," that is, one that centers around primary prevention and risk factor reduction and uses political and economic interventions such as the increased taxation of tobacco, lobbying, and increased media involvement, and public education to create and sustain broader health behavior change.

There is a need for rigorous research that is designed to evaluate the effectiveness of public health interventions (Glasgow et al. 1999, 2004). Although there is a large body of evidence that demonstrates the efficacy of behavioral interventions, the translation of research findings into practice is limited by the lack of useful models, incomplete methods, and the type and quality of data available (Glasgow et al. 2004). Much of what we have learned about the effectiveness of health interventions is limited by traditional disciplinary models and methods such as the linear cause-effect approach, while understanding the nature of the border and interventions to ameliorate its health and social problems requires a systems or ecological approach. What we need to know about the border, its problems, and program successes and failures is restricted by the kinds of questions we ask and the kinds of data we gather to answer them (Bruhn and Rebach 2007; Bruhn 2009; Bastida et al. 2008).

J. G. Bruhn, *Culture and Health Disparities*, SpringerBriefs in Public Health, DOI: 10.1007/978-3-319-06462-8_3, © The Author(s) 2014

3.2 Issues in Assessing the Effectiveness of Border Health Interventions

Data on health problems along the U.S.-Mexico border come primarily from 80 municipios in six Mexican states and 48 counties in four U.S. states. These data often lack common definitions and common data elements, may be gathered under different surveillance timelines and with different frequencies, and therefore have limited usefulness in planning and implementing interventions. The lack of data rigor can impede generalizability and distort important differences due to demography, culture, and/or disparities. For example, it is not possible to directly compare death rates in the U.S. and Mexico without considering that the majority population of Mexico is younger than the U.S. Similarly, the U.S. border region has lower rates of communicable diseases and some chronic diseases compared to the border region of Mexico, despite sharing some common risk factors. Without greater cross-border refinement of data content and coordination it will be difficult to identify and intervene in reducing risks and disparities. Available data and its current forms often determines *what* we study rather than build a data system focused on measurable variables that will yield data to fill existing knowledge gaps, and present new questions.

Available data not only influences what we research and evaluate but data are a product of the disciplinary perspective of the persons who gather the data. Researchers in medicine and public health have grown used to thinking about determinants of individual health, or more broadly about the health of populations, that they have neglected intermediate forms of social organization, such as communities and groups, especially the interaction between these levels. Different levels of analysis produce different data about health between the individual and population determinants as well as between different groups within a given population.

In recent literature public health researchers have reconsidered the contribution of social epidemiology. Many large scale studies have fallen short of expectations in identifying specific risk factors for disease onset and recurrence and many interventions to change individual high risk behaviors for certain diseases have been only minimally successful. Glass (2000) believes that these limitations are due to risk factors being viewed as discrete, voluntary, and individually modifiable lifestyle choices, detached from the social context in which behaviors arise. Syme (2004) stated that successes in smoking cessation have come about when they have been designed and implemented using a multipronged, multilevel, multidisciplinary approach. These approaches involve not only information but also regulations and laws, mass media programs, workplace rules, and better environmental engineering and design. Inevitably, he said, "We in public health need to think across disciplinary lines."

Much of public health epidemiological research and interventions have focused on individual-level factors in understanding the cause of between-population differences in disease rates and have promoted interventions that rely on change emerging from individual-level behavioral choices (Berkman 2004; Diez Roux 2004). Cohen and Syme (1985) explain, "an individual perspective...addresses the question of why one person gets sick while another person does not. A social perspective addresses the question of why one group or aggregation has a higher rate of disease than another…interventions can be viewed from both perspectives…the issue is not whether one approach is better than another but the usefulness of different approaches depending on their purpose."

Krieger (1994) discusses the limitations of what she calls "biomedical individualism" and challenges the current rigid distinction between individual and group-level analyses. She notes that there are health effects of groups that cannot be reduced to individual attributes. Corin (1994) states that individual health behavior cannot be fully understood unless the social and cultural context in which it is embedded is understood. The social context for studying the health behavior of groups is complex, dynamic, and needs to utilize diverse methods. Therefore, analyses of group behavior involves more than simply aggregating or averaging individual measures, or gathering observational data, or using multiple regression methods to control for individual-level confounding variables. When a determinant of health at the societal or group level of analysis is not confirmed as a risk factor in studies at the individual level of analysis, the societal finding is labeled an "ecological fallacy."

The health dynamics of populations or groups may involve factors that account for only a small part of individual variation in health and may escape detection. On the other hand, factors responsible for major differences in populations or groups may be so common that they go undetected in studies of individuals (Wilkinson 1996). The influence of social factors shared by most everyone in a population or group can only be detected by comparing different populations or groups. Important explanations for health differences between individuals do not explain differences within or between populations or groups.

Different levels of analyses produce different pictures of the determinants of health and different pictures of the effectiveness of health interventions. Studies of individuals lead to attempts to distinguish between people with and without some disease or social problem who all belong to the same population or social group. Comparisons of different groups with and without the same disease or social problem help to identify shared and unshared characteristics common to the problem, or help to identify common mechanisms by which the same problem is generated or prevented from occurring across different social and cultural contexts.

3.3 Examples of Gaps and Deficiencies in Intervention Research Along the U.S.-Mexico Border

3.3.1 Smoking Cessation

The leading causes of morbidity and mortality among Hispanics living in the U.S. are smoking related, specifically cardiovascular disease and lung cancer. Evidence suggests that the prevalence of smoking in this population will increase as Hispanics become more acculturated (Webb et al. 2010). Yet, of 12 intervention studies on smoking cessation that emerged since 1991 from a literature review and meta-analysis, only three were community-based interventions (Webb et al. 2010). While the strengths of these studies were their focus on a culturally specific approach, and the inclusion of a behavioral component, they were limited by high attrition, lack of comparison groups, short follow-up periods, unmatched treatment conditions, restricted age ranges, and nonrepresentative samples.

Future research should address these methodological limitations exploring the direct relationship between intervention and smoking status, as well as the interactive and mediating relationships between smoking and cultural variables. It is important that intervention designs recognize the significant heterogeneity among Hispanics that often have different language patterns and values. Multisite interventions with large and representative samples also increase the generalizability of findings. Future research and intervention studies should also consider the influence of acculturation, which has been shown to be related to tobacco initiation and treatment outcomes.

Reducing tobacco smoking can reduce morbidity and mortality, therefore future research and intervention activities have the potential of significantly impacting the health of border residents as well as Hispanics in the general U.S. population.

3.3.2 Preventing and Controlling Tuberculosis

Performance of TB control programs among the U.S.-Mexico binational population has not been characterized adequately in terms of prevention and treatment interventions because program evaluation requires sharing performance indicators especially: (1) targeted testing of specific high risk groups including persons with HIV infections and diabetes, immigrants, and medically underserved persons; (2) cooperation to strengthen diagnostic capabilities in Mexican border states, and (3) improved contact tracing by enhancing knowledge of social patterns of binational tracings and by developing a common contact protocol for the U.S. and Mexico (Lobato et al. 2001).

A Work Group Report (Lobato et al. 2001) proposed a multilevel approach to intervention in TB prevention and control. The Centers for Disease Control would work with state and local TB control programs and collaborate with public health and social scientists to develop and evaluate innovative methods for tracing, testing, and treating contacts of binational patients. Studies could then compare new strategies with past practices.

3.3.3 Knowledge-Action Gap in Diabetes

Type 2 diabetes (DM2) is the first cause of death in Mexico and the third leading cause in the U.S. A recent prevalence study that focused on a representative binational border population sample and used a common methodology found that 15 % of the U.S.-Mexico border population aged 18 years and older were affected by DM2 and 14 % were in the pre-diabetic stage (Cerqueira 2010). Evidence points to the need to create supportive environments for active lifestyles, increase access to healthy and affordable foods, improve outreach and access to quality health services, continue research to ascertain effective interventions, and increase surveillance along the border using a common methodology. Diabetes is a community issue. There is a need to identify elements of successful intervention programs such as using *promotoras* in outreach and education and community partnerships (Ingram et al. 2005).

3.3.4 HIV Prevention

Organista et al. (2004) reviewed and critiqued the HIV prevention outcome literature on Mexican migrants including U.S.-Mexico border inhabitants to identify gaps and recommend future research directions. They pointed to three overlapping complex approaches used to guide HIV prevention research. The first and predominant paradigm has been the behavioral approach based on theories of individual psychology that links HIV transmission primarily to behavioral and cognitive factors and co-factors such as drug use. A second approach builds on the first including social and cultural contexts that influence individual and group risk-related behaviors. A third approach focuses on structural, environmental, and social change issues. The authors point out that future research, service, and policy could be advanced if all three approaches were integrated.

Today, HIV prevention for Mexican migrants and related groups consists primarily of minimal and inconsistent HIV/AIDS education, condom promotion and distribution, HIV testing and counseling and support groups for affected individuals. For example, Moyer et al. (2008), found that only 38 % of injection drug users in Tijuana and 30 % in Ciudad Juarez had ever had an HIV test. Community-based organizations that provide health and social services have been found to be more effective in reaching Latinos than federal and state agencies because of their greater number of bilingual staff, volunteers, and culturally sensitive approaches to service delivery. While community-based interventions designed to improve knowledge of HIV transmissions are effective this approach is embedded in the individual cognitive model and does not address larger contextual aspects of HIV risk such as migration-related prostitution. Along the U.S.-Mexico border regional dynamics such as the drug and sex trade industries, tourism, transnationalism, and blurred sexual boundaries can result in significant HIV infections.

There is a need to increase our understanding of HIV risk, with an emphasis on sexuality and the ways that sex practices and beliefs vary across subgroups of migrants and border residents, and across different social, cultural, and relational contexts. Randomized controlled trends are difficult to implement with certain populations, but quasi-experimental research designs and mixed methods can be very useful. There is a need for conducting broader and more rigorous replications and/or modifications to better fit local research settings and subgroups of border migrants.

3.3.5 Environmental Issues

The North American Free Trade Agreement (NAFTA) and the presence of *maquiladoras* have intensified long-standing concerns about environmental health and hazardous waste issues along the U.S.-Mexico border. There are significant gaps in information about environmental quality. Current environmental quality monitoring focuses on air quality and surface water quality near large urban centers, but hazardous waste is not addressed (Carter et al. 1996). Specifically, environmental levels of pesticides and possible human exposure routes are not being targeted. Also, colonias' sources of water and their levels of hazardous wastes need monitoring.

Data gaps are a great problem because baseline information is necessary to better control and improve the identification of chemically induced diseases. To identify environmental health problems in the border region, the baseline incidence of disease must be determined in both U.S. and Mexican states. The influence of nutrition on chemical toxicity needs investigation. In the U.S. the border region is populated by a substantially lower socioeconomic class than in the rest of the country, a characteristic that is often limited to a higher incidence of nutritional deficiencies and more frequent exposure to infectious diseases. The incidence of lupus and the role of chemicals in its development needs investigation. Finally, analysis is needed of the data being generated at the border. Several state and federal agencies have established programs to analyze chemicals in air, water, and soil, but there are no efforts to analyze the data for trends, source of hazardous waste, or profiles of chemical waste. More targeted research is needed to evaluate the health impact of various wastes and waste treatment processes.

A U.S.-Mexico workshop was held to discuss many of the above issues. Recommendations were made, however, it was unclear to whom the recommendations should be directed (Carter et al. 1996). While there is heightened awareness of the environmental problems along the border and the data gaps that exist, progress is limited because it is undetermined who should take the lead, and how, and by whom, accountability will be assumed for solving these binational problems.

3.3.6 Mental Health

Discriminatory experiences have been found to be related to poor mental health outcomes and negative life changes among marginalized communities in the United States. Many socioeconomic and environmental conditions negatively influence the mental health of borderlanders including poverty, the lack of resources, drug trafficking, violence and immigration risks (Flores and Kaplan 2009). There is a paucity of studies of the mental health of borderlanders. Focus groups among Mexican Americans living along the southern border of Texas identified the lack of resources, knowledge about the causes and treatment for mental health problems, the importance of kinship among Hispanics, and the lack of providers who understood their needs as several key problems. Indicators of mental health issues encountered by borderlanders have been extracted from some U.S. prevalence studies that address the mental health of Latinos. In general, U.S.-born Latinos are at significantly higher risk for most psychiatric disorders compared to Latino immigrants and non-Latino whites. Traditional cultural practices have been suggested as a protective factor for Latino immigrants.

Cultural adaptations of evidence-based practices are necessary for treatment interventions to meet the needs of individuals, families, and communities, to impact treatment engagement, and to improve treatment outcomes. Even when borderlanders suffer from mental health problems they may not be able to access treatment due to their immigration status, fear, or knowledge of, and access to, resources. Furthermore, mental health care may not be a priority when individuals and families are faced with homelessness, poverty, hunger, violence and other problems related to daily survival. A significant amount of literature has pointed out that cultural values, language and level of acculturation are key variables in health care professionals and borderlanders experiencing biculturalism as the best model for positive mental health outcomes.

3.4 The Border Region as a Social System

The 2,000 mile long binational region shared by Mexico and the United States and its inhabitants is a social system. The region shares environmental, social, economic, cultural and health characteristics while retaining national sovereignty and different legal, political, and health systems, and public policies. Mexico and the United States are both independent and interdependent social systems. The actions and inactions of inhabitants on one side of the border have repercussions for inhabitants on the other side. The nature of this interrelationship is dynamic, complex, and constantly challenged by inadequate economic resources, changing politics, cultural and language differences and population growth.

A social system has many different levels of organization. In the case of Mexico and the U.S. the major levels are national, regional, state, county, and municipal. Ranging from the municipal level to the national level, each level is an incremental increase in social complexity. No level alone can completely explain the phenomenon occurring at that level, since all levels are interrelated. For example, factors at the national and regional levels are involved in the functioning of Mexican and U.S. communities. Each level explains only part of a total social system; for example, behavior at a higher or more complex level cannot be predicted from behavior at a lower level.

The goal of a social system is to achieve and maintain a balance between its parts so that it functions with relative cohesion and works constructively with other social systems. Activities that are defined as problems upset the cohesion or balance of a social system. Problem-solving and intervention is initiated to restore a sense of balance or equilibrium to an unbalanced one. The task of the problem solver is to learn how the system operates, especially what factors help it function in a positive manner, and assist with bringing about positive change. It is difficult, if not impossible to introduce change to one part of a system without affecting all parts of the system. The challenge is to learn what facilitates and inhibits balance in a social system with the intention of minimizing or controlling them so that the system can be enhanced and function in a preferred way (Bruhn and Rebach 2007).

A systems approach to solving and preventing border health problems has several advantages: (1) it can focus on several related problems simultaneously; (2) it identifies relationships where the cost of intervention is lowest and the effectiveness of intervention is highest; (3) it shifts the emphasis from quick-fix solutions to sustainable ones; (4) it includes options in solutions to adapt to change; (5) it helps maintain the integrity of complexity of a living system. Border health problems are simultaneously local and national; therefore, interventions at only one level will not bring about lasting solutions to problems (Bruhn and Rebach 2007). For example, an educational and outreach intervention to positively impact self-management behaviors for diabetes will be more sustainable and successful if it involves a consortium of providers at the community and county levels and an academic partner who provides technical assistance and objective evaluation (Ingram et al. 2005).

An example of the social systems approach is the U.S.-Mexico Border Diabetes Prevention and Control Project prevalence study (Cerqueira 2010). This study considered the U.S.-Mexico border area as an integral unit. Border counties and communities share more similarities among themselves than they do with their respective countries, especially in the case of U.S.-Mexico sister cities. This study used a representative binational border sample and a common methodology. The project has demonstrated the feasibility of effective, binational, interinstitutional, multi-disciplinary teamwork to achieve the common good of diabetes prevention and control.

3.5 Meso Level Interventions

The meso level has been a common intervention point in border health initiatives. People experience society in interaction with others at the meso level in a variety of organizations and social networks such as communities, organizations, neighborhoods, gangs, clubs, public agencies, corporate boards, and businesses. It is through these meso level structures that we find our identities and meet a variety of needs beyond those of the individual and family. These mediating structures link the macro and micro levels of a society. It is through the meso level that we can best intervene to solve problems. The meso level provides grassroots under-standing and data about the reality of everyday life. Indeed, to effect change in border health problems, there must be a buy-in and active support from citizens on both sides of the border. This is a challenge because culturally the same prob-lem may be perceived differently and/or economic and survival needs may give the same problem different priorities. Facilitators of communication such as community health workers or *promotoras* have been found to successfully serve as "bridges" between community members and health care services. An emerg-ing body of literature appears to support the unique role of the community worker and advocates in strengthening existing community networks for care, providing community members with support, education, and facilitating access to care (CDC Division of Diabetes Translation 2011; Steinfelt 2005; Balcazar et al. 2009; Elder et al. 2009; Hunter et al. 2004; Lara 1998; Ford et al. 1998; Brandon 1997).

Promotoras have been effective in providing appropriate context for inter-ventions in a wide range of problems from hypertension control (Balcazar et al. 2009), comprehensive preventive care (Hunter et al. 2004), depression (Waitzkin et al. 2011) to improving pesticide safety (Forster-Cox et al. 2007). The *promo-toras* is a meso level mechanism to create behavior change among individuals and families. The *promotoras*, however, are unlikely to effect significant systemic changes without assistance from macro level bureaucracies and agencies that shape health policy and allocate resources.

3.6 Data in the Intervention Process

3.6.1 Level of Analysis/Establishing a Need to Intervene

Interventions are only as effective as the data used to plan them. Although the U.S. and Mexico are two different geopolitical systems, the components or elements that make up the systems, e.g., national, regional, states, municipios, are similar. Therefore, there is some degree of comparability between, for example, a U.S. bor-der community and a Mexican municipios. Similarly, the 14 sister cities are both distinct social systems but together form a bi-cultural, geopolitical system unique to themselves. Understanding the differences and commonalities of the different levels of analysis is key to cross border interventions. For example, out of the 46 Mexican National Health Indicators and 25 United States Healthy Gente objectives there are 20 common measures. These represent priority areas for actions on health issues in the border region. However, differences in the national organization of health care service and data availability program objectives for both sides of the border are defined and refined by each county, state, or community (U.S.-Mexico Border Health Commission, Healthy Border 2010). While culturally unique inter-ventions are needed and respected, real progress will come in the future from

binational interventions, especially those at the community/municipios level of
analysis (Cerqueira 2009). Differences in data definitions and availability will need
to be overcome and a common binational data collection and retrieval bank will
need to be established if creditable, comparable, and consistent information for
planning and implementing interventions is to occur.

A common level of analysis used in intervention programs to date has been
those implemented at the community/municipios level. At the community level it
is usually easier to access information from subjects and involve them in establishing the need for an intervention as well as to implement programs and activities
that will directly translate to practice.

3.7 The Intervention Plan

After data has shown a need for an intervention it is useful to solicit the involvement of private and public collaborators and partners in planning the interventions
to insure that the plan will be culturally appropriate, meet needs, and be sustainable. Intervention plans usually falter if there is no clear goal at the onset and the
objectives and strategies for reaching the goal are not clear to all parties involved.
If there is no clearly agreed upon buy-in to the plan by all constituents it is likely
the plan will be plagued with set backs and will be unsustainable, when and if, it
is completed. A good intervention plan needs to be flexible, anticipate and plan for
change, yet not be too rigid about meeting the intended goal.

3.7.1 Baseline Data

Many interventions become scientifically unsound if they do not use a baseline of
data for planning an intervention. Ideally, the baseline data should include objective measures, but also include subjective data such as those from focus groups,
interviews, and surveys as well. Data collected in the course of carrying out the
intervention should be comparable to that in the baseline. In the case of a binational intervention the variables and their meanings and measurements should be
agreed upon if the baseline is to be common to both cultures.

3.7.2 Intervention Data

An intervention should be comprehensive in its measurements of the scope of its
impact. As such the evaluation of an intervention needs to collect both process
data and program data. Program data will provide evidence of the extent the intervention met its goal. Process data provides evidence the intervention plan was

executed according to plan with minimal bias and subject drop-out. Both levels of data are needed if the intervention is to be replicated with improvements. Both program and process data are important in bicultural interventions when the subtleties of language and culture can be factors in the success or failure of an intervention.

3.7.3 Follow-up Data

Some follow-up data are needed to gain insight into the sustainability of interventions. This is a special challenge for interventions on the U.S.-Mexico border where geographical mobility and anonymity are features of daily life. Short-term follow-up of less than 6 months is not an unreasonable goal, long-term follow-ups of 1 year or longer are a challenge. Working at the community level enables follow-ups as it is more likely *promotoras* would be able to learn and access the social networks of small communities. Follow-ups need to be part of the recruitment of participants for any intervention, especially a commitment of their willingness to provide brief access to them.

3.7.4 Translation to Practice

Binational, bicultural interventions are especially challenged to be practical, useful, and to fit into one's culture as comfortably as possible if follow through and lifestyle changes are a goal. Indeed, any intervention threatens one's values and their prioritization in one's life. Part of the intervention could incorporate the opportunity to discuss the impact of an intervention on one's self, family and extended family. This would also provide the opportunity for interveners to learn more about the personal and familial aspects of health behavior change and provide insights about how border residents can be more fully engaged in making health choices.

3.8 Sharing Data

There is a need to replicate well-designed intervention studies to improve generalizability such as the use of *promotoras*, and evaluate and compare various intervention models at different levels of analysis. More intervention studies need to be designed cross-culturally so that partnerships and shared resources can be used to enhance sustainability on both sides of the border. Border centers of excellence can facilitate the establishment of shared databases to reduce duplication, costs, and personnel and initiate projects that will build on the capacity of successful models.

3.8.1 Cross-Border Networks

Although cross-border cooperation can be a rational approach to developing cross-border interventions, these collaborations are complex (Woodrow Wilson Center 2009). There are different levels of collaboration ranging from verbal agreements to carrying out a short-term project to committing money and personnel toward sustainability (Collins 2012). Also, the ability of partners to overcome language and cultural differences and who are similarly motivated is key. Lara-Valencia (2011) has termed this the "thickening" of the U.S.-Mexico Border.

3.9 Evaluating Interventions to Reduce Healthcare Disparities

The literature on evaluating interventions is diverse and complicated largely because of differing methodology, especially in identifying target groups for interventions and appropriate study designs for evaluating interventions. Cooper et al. (2002) highlight some of the limitations of previous studies. In most studies only a limited number of health determinants have been targeted. Second, many interventions have not been described in sufficient detail to be adapted or replicated in other settings. Third, only a small number of studies have been tailored for ethnic minority groups. Fourth, many interventions have not used models that account for barriers to changing provider behavior. Many studies have used small samples, failed to use control groups and/or had short follow-up periods. Fifth, most interventions have focused on healthcare services and health behaviors.

To remedy some of these deficiencies and focus evaluation research, the Robert Wood Johnson Foundation (RWJF), in 2005, created a nationally competitive initiative to provide grants to fund the evaluation of healthcare interventions that hold promise for reducing racial and ethnic disparities and improve healthcare for minorities. The effort was called *The Finding Answers Program*. Eleven grants were funded from an initial pool of 177 brief proposals. Most of these proposals targeted African-Americans and Hispanics. The majority of proposals were directed toward adults in urban areas (Schlotthauer et al. 2008).[1]

While the RWJF program is not the only effort, it is the largest and most focused effort in the U.S. to date. The interventions most commonly proposed were organization-level and patient-level projects (Chin et al. 2007). These results are consistent with the literature that identified multicomponent interventions targeting different leverage points, nurse-led case management in the context of wider systems change, culturally tailored quality improvement, and community health

---

[1] Despite an accumulating literature concerned with racial and ethnic disparities in children's health, there have been few published studies of interventions that have been successful in eliminating these disparities. See Flores (2009).

workers, as showing promise. Successful interventions need to be disseminated and replicated in a variety of populations and settings (Schlotthauer et al. 2008).

3.10 Factors Associated with Success

Several studies have reported improved health of disadvantaged groups (Gepkens and Gunning-Schepers 1996; Arblaster et al. 1996). Ensuring community commitment and input from community leaders and stakeholders have led to success. When community leaders and members participate in designing and conducting needs assessment, delivering the intervention, and evaluating the intervention and its impact, they have proven to contribute to intervention success. Multidisciplinary investigator teams and multifaceted approaches are other strategies that have led to success. Also, cultural appropriateness and competence of the interventionists have been critical to the success of interventions (Cooper et al. 2002).

3.11 Summary

The U.S.-Mexico border region presents many challenges to the typical model of intervention in public health. A social systems approach which links individual, group, and population levels of data seems appropriate for understanding how and why micro and macro factors interact to produce positive and negative health effects. A systems approach provides a holistic understanding of risks and protective factors that give rise to certain health behaviors. Moreover, a systems approach provides insights into how health interventions can be effective in creating behavioral change and increase sustainability.

The social systems approach embraces cultural uniqueness and differences, and as such, is a useful model for health interventions along the U.S.-Mexico border. Many interventions have fallen short of the usual process followed in intervention studies, hence, generalizability and reproducibility are compromised. Future data needs include sharing databases and establishing collaborations so that more interventions can be carried out with greater scientific rigor and yield stronger applications to practice.

References

Arblaster, L., Lambert, M., Entwisle, V., et al. (1996). A systematic review of the effectiveness of health service interventions aimed at reducing inequalities in health. *Journal of Health Services Research and Policy, 1*(2), 93–103.

Balcazar, H. G., Byrd, T. L., Ortiz, M., Tondapu, S. R., & Chavez, M. (2009). A randomized community intervention to improve hypertension control among Mexican Americans: Using the Promotoras de Salud community outreach model. *Journal of Health Care for the Poor and Underserved, 20*(4), 1079–1094.

Bastida, E., Brown, H. S., & Pagan, J. A. (2008). Persistent disparities in the use of health care along the U.S.-Mexico border: An ecological perspective. *American Journal of Public Health, 98*(11), 1987–1995.

Berkman, L. F. (2004). Introduction: Seeing the forest and the trees—From observation to experiments in social epidemiology. *Epidemiological Reviews, 26*(1), 2–6.

Brandon, J. E. (1997). Health promotion efforts along the U.S.-Mexico border. In J. G. Bruhn & J. E. Brandon (Eds.), *Border health: Challenges for the United States and Mexico* (pp. 163–179). New York: Garland Publishing Inc.

Bruhn, J. G. (2009). *The group effect: Social cohesion and health outcomes.* New York: Springer.

Bruhn, J. G., & Rebach, H. M. (2007). *Sociological practice: Intervention and social change.* New York: Springer.

Carter, D. E., Pena, C., Varady, R., & Suk, W. A. (1996). Environmental health and hazardous waste issues related to the U.S.-Mexico border. *Environmental Health Perspectives, 104*, 590–594.

CDC Division of Diabetes Translation and Division of Adult and Community Health, Community Health Worker and Promotora de Salud Workgroup Members. (2011). *Community Health Workers/Promotoras de Salud: Critical connections in communities.* Retrieved January 15, 2011, from http://www.cdc.gov/diabetes/projects/comm.htm.

Cerqueira, M. T. (2009). Center of Excellence, Pan American Health Organization (PAHO), U.S.-Mexico Border Office. Retrieved January 25, 2011, from www.borderhealth.org/border_models_of_excellence.php?curr=bhc_initiatives.

Cerqueira, M. T. (2010). Bridging the knowledge-action gap in diabetes along the U.S.-Mexico border. *Revista Panamericana de Salud Publica/Pan American Journal of Public Health, 28*(3), 139–140.

Chin, M. H., Walters, A. E., & Huang, E. S. (2007). Interventions to reduce racial and ethnic disparities in health care. *Medical Care Research Review, 64*(5 Suppl), 75–285.

Cohen, S., & Syme, S. L. (1985). *Social support and health* (p. 19). New York: Academic Press.

Collins, K. (2012). *Finding sustainability in the U.S.-Mexico borderlands: A look toward democracy and the public interest.* Paper presented at Public Administration Theory Conference, South Padre Island, TX, May 18–21.

Cooper, L. A., Hill, M. H., & Powe, N. R. (2002). Designing and evaluating interventions to eliminate racial and ethnic disparities in health care. *Journal of General Internal Medicine, 17*(6), 477–486.

Corin, E. (1994). The social and cultural matrix of health and disease. In R. G. Evans, M. L. Barer, & T. R. Marmor (Eds.), *Why are some people healthy and others not? The determinants of health of populations* (pp. 93–132). New York: Walter de Gruyter.

Diez Roux, A. V. (2004). The study of group-level factors in epidemiology: Rethinking variables, study designs, and analytical approaches. *Epidemiologic Reviews, 26*(1), 104–111.

Elder, J. P., Ayala, G. X., Parra-Medina, D., & Talavera, G. A. (2009). Health communication in the Latino community: Issues and approaches. *Annual Review of Public Health, 30*, 227–251.

Flores, G. (2009). Devising, implementing, and evaluating interventions to eliminate healthcare disparities in minority children. *Pediatrics, 124*(Suppl 3), 5214–5223.

Flores, L., & Kaplan, A. (Eds.). (2009). *Addressing the mental health problems of border and immigrant youth.* Los Angeles, CA: National Center for Child Traumatic Stress.

Ford, L. A., Barnes, M. D., Crabtree, R. D., & Fairbanks, J. (1998). Boundary spanners: Las Promotoras in the borderlands. In J. G. Power & T. Byrd (Eds.), *U.S.-Mexico border health: Issues for regional and migrant populations* (pp. 141–164). Thousand Oaks, CA: Sage.

Forster-Cox, S. C., Mangadu, T., Jacquez, B., & Corona, A. (2007). The effectiveness of the promotora (community health worker) model of intervention for improving pesticide safety in U.S./Mexico border homes. *Californian Journal of Health Promotion, 5*(1), 62–75.

Ganster, P., & Lorey, D. E. (2008). *The U.S.-Mexico border in the 21st century* (2nd ed.). Lanham, MD: Rowman & Littlefield Publishers.

Gepkens, A., & Gunning-Schepers, L. J. (1996). Interventions to reduce socioeconomic health differences: A review of the international literature. *European Journal of Public Health, 6*, 218–226.

Glass, T. A. (2000). Psychosocial intervention. In L. Berkman & I. Kawachi (Eds.), *Social epidemiology* (pp. 267–305). New York: Oxford University Press.

Glasgow, R. E., Klesges, L. M., Dzewaltowski, D. A., Bull, S. S., & Estrabrooks, P. (2004). The future of health behavior change research: What is needed to improve translation of research into health promotion practice. *Annals of Behavioral Medicine, 27*(1), 3–12.

Glasgow, R. E., Vogt, T. M., & Boles, S. M. (1999). Evaluating the public health impact of health promotion interventions: The RE-AIM framework. *American Journal of Public Health, 89*, 1322–1327.

Homedes, N., & Ugalde, A. (2003). Globalization and health at the United States-Mexico border. *American Journal of Public Health, 93*(12), 2016–2022.

Homedes, N., & Ugalde, A. (2009, October 1–5). Shaping health reform for the U. S.-Mexico border region. *Texas Business Review.*

Hunter, J. B., de Zapien, J. G., Papenfuss, M., Fernandez, M. L., Meister, J., & Giuliano, A. R. (2004). The impact of a "Promotora" on increasing routine chronic disease prevention among women aged 40 and older at the U.S.-Mexico border. *Health Education & Behavior, 31*(4), 185–285.

Ingram, M., Gallegos, G., & Elenes, J. (2005). Diabetes is a community issue: The critical elements of a successful outreach and education model on the U.S.-Mexico border. *Preventing Chronic Disease, 2*(1), A15.

Kozel, C. T., Hubbell, A. P., Dearing, J. W., Kane, W. M., et al. (2006). Exploring agenda-setting for Healthy Border 2010: Research directions and methods. *Californian Journal of Health Promotion, 4*(1), 141–161.

Krieger, N. (1994). Epidemiology and the web of causation: Has anyone seen the spider? *Social Science and Medicine, 39*(7), 887–903.

Lara, J. (1998). Health outreach programs in the colonias of the U.S.-Mexico border. In J. G. Power & T. Byrd (Eds.), *U.S.-Mexico border health: Issues for regional and migrant populations* (pp. 208–214). Thousand Oaks, CA: Sage.

Lara-Valencia, F. (2011). The "thickening" of the U.S.-Mexico Border: Prospects for cross-border networking and cooperation. *Journal of Borderlands Studies, 26*(3), 251–264.

Lobato, M. N., in collaboration with Work Group members. (2001). Preventing and controlling tuberculosis along the U.S.-Mexico border. *MMWR, 50*(RR1), 1–2.

Moyer, L. B., Brouwer, K. C., Brodine, S. K., Ramos, R., Lozada, R., Cruz, M. F., et al. (2008). Barriers and missed opportunities to HIV testing among injection users in two Mexico-U.S. border cities. *Drug Alcohol Review, 27*(1), 39–45.

Organista, K. C., Carrillo, H., & Ayala, G. (2004). HIV prevention with Mexican migrants: Review, critique, and recommendations. *JAIDS Journal of Acquired Immune Deficiency Syndromes, 37*, S227–S239.

Schlotthauer, A., Badler, A., Cook, S. C., Perez, D. J., & Chin, M. H. (2008). Evaluating interventions to reduce health care disparities: An RWJF program. *Health Affairs, 27*(2), 568–573.

Steinfelt, V. E. (2005). The border health strategic initiative from a community perspective. *Preventing Chronic Disease.* http://www.cdc.gov/pcd/issues/2005/jan/040077.htm.

Syme, S. L. (2004). Social determinants of health: The community as an empowered partner. *Preventing Chronic Disease, 1*(1), 1–5.

U.S.-Mexico Border Health Commission. (2003). *Healthy border 2010: An agenda for improving health on the United States-Mexico border.* A conference held at New Mexico State University, Las Cruces, October 2–4, 2003.

U.S.-Mexico Border Health Commission. (2010). *Health disparities and the U.S.-Mexico border: Challenges and opportunities.* A White paper, October 25. El Paso, TX.

Waitzkin, H., Getrich, C., Heying, S., Rodriguez, L., et al. (2011). Promotoras as mental health practitioners in primary care: A multi-method study as an intervention to address contextual sources of depression. *Journal of Community Health, 36*(2), 316–331.

Webb, M. S., Rodriguez-Esquivel, D., & Baker, E. A. (2010). Smoking cessation interventions among Hispanics in the United States: A systematic review and mini meta-analysis. *American Journal of Health Promotion, 25*(2), 109–118.

Wilkinson, R. G. (1996). Unhealthy societies: The affections of inequality (pp. 1–9 and 12–21). New York: Routledge.

Woodrow Wilson International Center for Scholars. (2009). Mexico Institute. *The United States and Mexico: Towards a strategic partnership.* A report of four working groups on U.S.-Mexico Relations. Woodrow Wilson Center, Mexico Institute.

Chapter 4
Ethical Issues in Health Interventions Across Contexts and Cultures

4.1 Introduction

Public health interventions have a long history (Kass 2001). Generally public health seeks to improve the well-being of communities through social actions. It is critical that the intervention's design and implementation are socially and culturally effective, useful, replicative, and cost-effective. In short, public health interventions aim to change behaviors and lifestyles that are detrimental to longevity and the quality of life. In order to accomplish public health goals, groups, communities, and nations need to be receptive to, and implement, programs whose effects may confront their health values and/or how those values are practiced. Public health programs should embrace evaluation so that feedback can be used to further enhance interventional outcomes. The methods and techniques used in evaluation are important in analyzing outcomes for program betterment.

Interventions create change. Change is often controversial because it is broad, complex, and, no matter how well it is controlled, its consequences are not fully known. Interventions are also political; they have consequences for public policy (Oliver 2006). It is well known, for example, that social, cultural, and economic factors cause substantial inequalities in health. It is argued by some that inequalities are unfair, affect everyone, are avoidable, and are cost ineffective (Woodward and Kawachi 2000).

4.1.1 Cultural Leverage

Fisher et al. (2007) have suggested that interventions using cultural leverage can be used to narrow social disparities in healthcare. Cultural leverage, which includes cultural competence, has shown promise as a strategy for improving healthcare (Beach et al. 2005; Brach and Fraser 2000). Interventions that are responsive to the cultural needs of a community are more likely to be effective (Castro et al. 2004; Gorin et al. 2012; Holmes et al. 2008).

J. G. Bruhn, *Culture and Health Disparities*, SpringerBriefs in Public Health,
DOI: 10.1007/978-3-319-06462-8_4, © The Author(s) 2014

Interveners attempt to develop interventions that will succeed; that is, have a beneficial outcome for the participants in the intervention. Hopefully, others can replicate successful interventions with minor changes. However, behavioral and lifestyle interventions are difficult to design and implement, resulting in a range of outcomes and thus a paradoxical literature. Baranowski and Hearn (1997) pointed out that many articles do not provide sufficient detail about an intervention for it to be replicated, and often provide little rationale for selecting the form and nature of the interventions used. In addition, process evaluation is absent in most articles and thus, the reader must infer why an intervention did or did not work. The literature on interventions often conveys an unclear and conflicting picture of the results of evaluation.

4.2 Definitions

Several key terms set the stage for this discussion. Webster defined *interventions* "to come between points in time or events, to maintain or alter a condition or prevent or compel an action," outcome as "something that follows as a result or consequence," and success as a "degree of measure of succeeding, favorable or desired outcome." Loewy (1989) defined *ethics* as "acts that affect others." *Participants* are people who volunteer for intervention programs, activities, or clinical trials.

4.3 Conditions of Interventions

4.3.1 Intervention Is a Process

Intervention is viewed as a discrete set of behaviors, activities, or actions that are planned and designed by an intervener and conveyed to a participant at a given point. Periodic assessments or measurements determine how the intervention has changed or modified the participants' physical, psychological, or social behavior. Interventions can take place or be administered more than once. Follow-up to assess changes may be undertaken after the intervention. Assessments or measurements during and at the end of a specified time are used to determine the success or failure of the intervention.

What is lacking in this scenario is an appreciation that intervention is a process. The intervener, participant, and the intervention are all moving targets. Because they change over time, they are not the same at the end as they were at the onset of the intervention. Interveners plan interventions to be similar to minimize bias; however, interventions are implemented by people who themselves change. Therefore, interventions are only approximations, not ideal replications. Intervention is influenced by change, hence, without a detailed monitoring of the process of an intervention, it is not possible to determine the effect of serendipity or unexpected influences on outcome. This is a significant omission in most published reports (Table 4.1).

Table 4.1 Ethical issues to be considered in designing, implementing, and evaluating health interventions across cultures

- *Representation of personnel*—be certain that the project personnel represent the social and demographic characteristics of the population involved and that these parties have input
- *Strengthen values*—be aware of the beliefs and values of the populations involved so that conflicts and misunderstandings are prevented
- *Set incremental goals*—set both realistic short term and long-term incremental goals so that the populations involved feel neither overwhelmed or under-challenged
- *Preventing failure of an intervention*—budget planning and resource allocation needs to precede interventions
- *Identify the cultural supports and constraints for change*—be aware of the politics surrounding the intervention so that it does not become the scapegoat for a failed intervention
- *Responsibility for follow-up*—specify who, what, and when, and how both short and long term follow-up will be carried out at the completion of the intervention
- *Establish who and how cultural power for decision-making will be made*
- *What are the cultural values that determine* the form(s) for measuring change in disparities?
- *How will on-going leadership,* data analysis, and translation of findings be shared across cultures?
- *How will community support be created* and maintained throughout the intervention?

4.3.2 Intervention Is an Intrusion into Value Systems

When professionals attempt to change situations, they confront people with their values. The proposed change is "known" by the professional to be the best for the participant or client. Clients also "know" what is best for them. The process of "knowing" involves the direct or intuitive assessment of values. The strength or depth of the commitment that the professional and client have to their values, and the congruence between their values, will determine whether intervention is possible, and if so, the ease with which it can be carried out. Professionals often assume that the interventions they propose are "right," and that the rejection of an intervention by a client means that the client is not serious about change. Professionals' assessments of why some clients reject interventions or why particular interventions were not successful are value judgments. Value conflicts are rarely mentioned as reasons for failure (Bruhn and Rebach 1996).

4.3.3 Intervention Is Based on a Relationship of Trust and Expectations

Irrespective of whether the participant in an intervention is a child, adult, family, or community, a professional relationship must be established between the intervener and the participant. In this relationship, intervener and participant share information about the risks and benefits of participating in the intervention, the duties and responsibilities of the participant (i.e., adherence to the protocol) are outlined, and both parties sign an informed consent agreement.

It is important that participants see the intervener involved throughout the intervention process. Often, however, the person who recruits the participant is someone of rank and status whom the participant rarely sees. The people with whom the participant interacts often are technicians with whom the participant can establish only perfunctory relationships.

Interventions can be rigid in design and paternalistically administered, or they can be negotiable and make allowances for the participant's autonomy. How an intervention is structured and monitored depends on whether it is a treatment (clinical) or preventive (education) intervention. Clinical interventions tend to be more structured than educational ones.

4.3.4 Intervention Is Not an All or None Action

Interveners want their interventions to succeed. Participants are similarly motivated, especially if the intervention is a treatment for a disease. Sometimes interveners focus so intensely on the intervention and its effects that other factors in the participant's life are ignored or forgotten as intervening variables. It is tempting for interveners to assume that they identified and accounted for the pertinent intervening variables, but some unexpected ones may emerge in the process of implementing the intervention. This is why it is important to consider participants as individuals as well as members of a group. The effects of interventions may not apply uniformly to all participants. On the other hand, participants in successful interventions may share characteristics with participants in unsuccessful interventions. The outcome may be determined by who and how many participants are recruited and their reasons for participating. For example, paying volunteers may not increase the likelihood that an intervention will be successful.

4.4 Ethical Issues in Intervention Outcomes

4.4.1 The Goals of the Intervention

Jenkins (1992) said that the ultimate purpose of all health interventions is to enhance the quality of life. He argues that judging the quality of any health intervention requires measuring the post intervention health-related quality of life. Similarly, Schalock (1995) noted that the intervention outcome needs to be valued by the participant; therefore, the purpose of the intervention must be clear in order to recruit participants. Participants want to know when they will see evidence of change resulting from an intervention; the type and extent of their duties and responsibilities as participants; any trade-offs they might have to make in their attitudes, behavior, and lifestyles; and the necessary extent of their commitments of time and energy.

The goals of clinical (treatment focused) interventions are usually easier to define and may have observable and quantifiable outcomes (e.g., the efficacy of a new drug). The goals of educational interventions are value-laden, often less quantifiable, and may take several years for results to become observable.

Fraser (1989) suggested that health professionals do not intervene to "solve problems." Real solutions, he says, are achieved by rearranging attitudes and values. Mediation is an example of an intervention that often results in the growth of the participants' ability to manage the potential for conflict positively and create opportunities for creative problem solving. A successful intervention could be said to be one from which participants emerge believing that they can manage their values more effectively. This supports Baranowski and Nader's (1985) observations that family dynamics is a better indicator of compliance than is family structure in family and child compliance regimens. How a family manages itself is a better indicator of how it might benefit from an intervention than do objective family characteristics or structure.

A failure to involve or empower individuals, families, and communities in the design and implementation of interventions will affect the outcome of the intervention. The more participants buy into and share the goals of an intervention, the more likely they are to assist in its success. The degree of the participants' involvement with the design and implementation of the intervention will vary with the goal of the intervention. Broad outcomes, such as making major changes in lifestyle, likely will require more input from participants than would changes for the treatment of a specific disease. In some cases, too much involvement by participants may bias results and limit the generalizability of results; that is, interventions that are designed only for the needs of a particular group may not be applicable to other groups. Kline (1999) noted that cultural factors are important in determining the goals of an intervention because cultural factors help to shape health attitudes and behavior, and affect people's responses to changes that affect their health status (Kline 1999).

4.4.2   Context of the Intervention and its Sustainability

Foeyt et al. (1981) stated that, although behavior change has been obtained during the course of an intervention, the behavior often reverts to baseline levels after discontinuation of the intervention. A motivated family member may encounter resistance from the rest of the family when attempting to involve them in a behavior change. Successful outcomes have been reported in parent-child and in couples' weight loss programs when positive reinforcement is provided by parents or a significant other. Positive support has also been found to be important in abstaining from smoking and in maintaining blood pressure control. Heller et al. (1990) noted that most individuals achieve esteem through the practice of role behaviors in reciprocal relationships. If they are to be sustained over time, interventions should be embedded in people's usual social networks.

It is important that there be some continuity between the context of the intervention and the participant's social and cultural context following the intervention. Heller and his colleagues (1990) stated that it is difficult for individuals to change their behaviors or adopt new behaviors without appropriate social contexts that reinforce these changes. Baranowski (1997) discussed the problems in the sustainability of interventions in family dietary practices. Sustainability should be addressed with participants in the intervention from the onset so that their expectations of the intervention are realistic and there will be less chance, after they are removed from the supportive structure of the project, that they will revert to former habits.

4.4.3 Feedback to Participants

The design of interventions—the rules and responsibilities for participants and their opportunity for input—can range in their degree of structuredness. Most interventions are not negotiable because it is important that participants follow a similar protocol to minimize the effects of intervening variables.

Feedback during an intervention is extremely important. Participants need to know results of tests, "how they are doing," and receive encouragement. Interveners, in turn, need to know how pleased or displeased participants are with the protocol or regimen and be willing to make modifications to minimize drop-outs. Often, there is no ongoing exchange of information between the intervener and participant. Tailoring interventions to fit individuals, families, and communities is possible, depending upon the intervention and its goals, but "making the intervention more palatable" is no guarantee that the participant will stick with changes. Baranowski and Hearn noted that evaluations of interventions must assess whether programs were implemented as designed, and if not, why not, and what characteristics of the participants were related to the level of compliance achieved.

4.4.4 Timing of the Intervention

People choose to participate in interventions for a variety of reasons. Their degree of readiness or motivation to participate is related to other events in their lives. There is a "right time" for everyone to engage. Potential participants in an intervention may decline to participate because they are coping with "too much" change in their lives, or they may choose to participate because they have reached a status quo or dead end with respect to other alternatives. People choose to participate in interventions because they hope that by doing so they will improve their lives. Altruistic motives, meeting new friends, peer pressure, or the desire to look good to others may also be contributing factors. Knowledge about why the participant chooses to join a change effort is valuable information for the intervener because it may provide insights about the person's plans and ability to continue with the implemented changes following the intervention.

It is also helpful for participants to know why a particular intervention is offered at this time. Is it because the intervener received a research grant, is this a new or ongoing program in a university, or has the intervener been chosen to participate in a national clinical trial dealing with a specific disease? Participants need to know the level of interest and the commitment of the intervener. This information is valuable to participants in their assessment of risks and benefits, and in their assessment of how committed the intervener is to the project.

For example, medical centers offer the opportunity for HIV and AIDS patients to join clinical trials to test the efficacy of new drugs. These opportunities offer hope to patients for an improvement in their illness, but also the ability to interact with the same clinic personnel who provide a degree of social support to the patient in coping with the devastation and uncertainty AIDS creates in their lives. When the clinical trial ends or clinic personnel leave, patients may also leave searching for new opportunities for cure and support. Thus, patients' eagerness to participate in an intervention is often driven by socioemotional needs that accompany their illness and their prior illness experience (Bruhn 1994).

Rolland (1994), in his work with families, stated that the typology and time phases of illness, combined with an understanding of individual and family lifecycles, offer a useful framework for timing interventions. Rather than suggest automatic visits or check-ups every few months, Rolland used important lifecycle and illness transitions as a guide for timing consultations and brief interventions. Families can be educated to anticipate changes, recognize signs of the need for help, and request intervention in a more preventive manner. Brown (1991) similarly pointed out that major disruptions and transitions in the family are opportunities for change, but clients must determine when a change is necessary and assume responsibility for being the agent of change.

4.4.5 Are Drop-Outs Failures?

There is no debate that people who volunteer for research and other kinds of projects tend to differ from other members of the general population (Rosenthal and Rosnow 1975). Among volunteers, those who "adhere" to regimens have been found to differ from volunteers who do not adhere to regimens (Masur 1981). Gochman (1997) suggested that the words "compliance" and "adherence" are out of vogue and a new term is needed for people who volunteer for research and intervention projects and stick with them. Furthermore, all people who stick with a project are not necessarily successful in achieving its goals. That does not necessarily mean that participants who drop out of interventions prematurely, or who do not achieve the intervener's goals, are failures. Participants have goals for themselves, which they may or may not vocalize to project personnel. A person whose own goals have been met may not see a reason to continue in the intervention. Life situations change and unforeseen events may arise, making it difficult for a participant to continue in a project. Some interventions may confront participants with choices they find uncomfortable or are unwilling to make, and therefore, they drop out. Masur (1981) suggested that "compliance" can be improved by educating the client to better understand the instructions and the regimen in interventions. But, as Di Matteo (1997) suggested, nonadherence is an interactional problem, a reflection of poor communication between the intervener and participant. In addition, the paternalistic approach that the words "compliance" and "adherence" invoke conflict with current attempts to increase client autonomy in decision-making about one's health.

4.4.6 The Limits of Shared Commitment

Interventions succeed or fail based on the strength of shared commitments. The intervener must "sell" participants on the goals of the intervention. Participants must "buy" into the intervention not only in terms of how it might benefit them personally, but also to its broader effect on others. The intervener must be clear with the participants about what kind of change, and its extent, is expected. Participants, in turn must buy into the process of change and what it entails for them. Legally, this is done through the informed consent form that both the intervener and the participant sign. And, the structure or "rules" surrounding participant's involvement in the project is usually spelled out before participants' agree to become involved. Yet it is the psychological or emotional "buy in" that is often not totally clarified up front. Some interveners request participants to draft contracts so that both the intervener and participant have quantifiable measures of the degree of success reached at the end of the intervention. A contract helps to make expectations explicit and minimize misunderstanding. All of these efforts help in structuring the shared commitment.

Yet, there is a social aspect of shared commitment that is not easily quantifiable and that may change as participation in the intervention proceeds. This element can surprise interveners when a participant suddenly drops out or becomes resistant. Sometimes interventions look and feel good at the onset, but after involvement, participants become dissatisfied. The more interveners and their staff know the participants as individuals, the less likely there will be a problem. There should be an ongoing determination of individual participants' resilience and commitment to personal change (Rolf and Johnson 1999). This can be done informally so that participants do not feel that they are being challenged or their motivation questioned.

Interveners can ask participants to change one behavior, several, or their complete lifestyle. It is likely that changing one behavior requires minimal effort, whereas a lifestyle change might be overwhelming. There is a vast difference in the degree of commitment participants will likely make to these two extreme alternatives. Interveners should not ask too much or too little of participants in interventions. On the other hand, participants need to have realistic expectations of the outcomes from their participation; they have to accept the premises of the intervention, personalize them, and be committed to personally changing aspects of their lives. Interveners and participants should communicate frequently and directly to reaffirm their shared commitments to the goals of the intervention.

4.4.7 Iatrogenic Issues

One would expect interventions that are developed and implemented to be "good" for the participants. Because the literature suggests that eating the right foods, getting sufficient exercise, refraining from smoking, controlling stress, and having a strong social support system are conductive to good health and well-being and may help to prevent certain diseases and promote longevity, it could be assumed that the intervener supports this view and attempts to convince participants to change their lifestyles to adopt more healthy ones. Some participants may not be able to change more than one behavior successfully, others may change several behaviors, but extensive changes may not be within the motivation reach of the majority of participants. Participants who are not successful in reaching the intervener's goal for them may feel that they have failed, and indeed, after the intervention, may give up the changes they have already made. Thus, the expectations of the intervener may be unrealistic for some participants. Interventions could cause some participants to become anxious and depressed and to give up trying to achieve a healthier life.

In the case of low-income participants, dietary interventions, such as more frequent consumption of fruits, vegetables, and low-fat foods may tax the family budget unrealistically. Ethnic minority individuals and families who reject traditional foods in favor of typical American foods could become objects of ridicule or become socially isolated. As Paul pointed out several decades ago, "health programs should start with people as they are and the community as it is" (Paul 1955). Each group has its own social and physical environment. Groups cannot be evaluated on a single scale; each is a product of numerous historical and situational factors. It is difficult to change those cultural features that serve as symbols and control the motivations of individuals, even in apparently simple matters.

4.4.8 Who the Intervener Is?

Many family and community health interventions are carried out by a variety of healthcare professionals. Participants may not see the same personnel at each of their periodic visits. Depending on the intervention, personnel may represent a variety of disciplines; therefore, participants may have difficulty in developing strong identification and loyalty to the project or program and confusion about who they can question about their progress. This is particularly true for large interventions with extensive staff.

It may matter to some participants that they talk to a person with the power or status that a white coat conveys; however, when everyone they see wears a white coat, they may be confused about who to confide in or who has decision-making authority with respect to them.

The degree of rapport established between the participant and the health professional responsible for the intervention influences whether the participants will stick to and follow through with behaviors learned during the intervention. The attitudes and behaviors of the caretakers toward the participants can also affect attrition. Participants are volunteers and altruistic and expect appreciation for their time and for sharing information about themselves.

4.5 Reevaluating Success in Interventions

Success in interventions is usually assessed by determining whether the difference in the degree of change in the experimental group compared to that of the control group is statistically significant. Was the change in the predicted direction? Did the intervention have a sufficient number of participants to warrant generalization to the general population? Is the intervention replicable? Broader concerns include issues such as, whether the intervention was more beneficial than harmful to the participants and how the public will benefit from this experiment.

An intervention may be unsuccessful for a cohort but beneficial for some individuals in the cohort. Similarly, an intervention for a cohort may be deemed successful, but fail to benefit some individuals in the cohort. Interventions that are not totally successful or unsuccessful may attain degrees of both. We often miss the secrets of success and failure because we fail to examine the individuals who differed from the majority to see what factors or characteristics contributed to their success or failure. Interventions are often on a fast track to determine whether or not a particular array of strategies induces change. These strategies are usually developed with an eye toward producing results that fit the principal investigators' definition of success. When input from participants is absent, their definition of what success is will also be absent.

4.5.1 What Contributes to Successful Interventions?

We know less than we should about unsuccessful interventions because reports about them are not published or, if they are, provide insufficient introspection about what went wrong (and what went right) to help the reader know what to avoid (or do) in a replication. Therefore, it is not surprising that few interventions are replicated. Seemingly, every investigator wants to be a pioneer in developing a successfully acclaimed intervention. Interventions and the details of their formats and strategies become as protected as patents and copyrights.

Oldenburg et al. (1999) pointed out that contemporary health promotion research does not appear to be focusing on the social and environmental contexts of health behaviors or using broader strategies in implementing interventions. In their critique of the published literature, Oldenburg and colleagues also state that many health promotion research findings are difficult to apply in real-life settings, hence practitioners either find that academic research is not relevant to many of the health issues they face or that there is insufficient information about how to use the strategies for change. Some interventions fail because they are too focused and either ignore or forget the fact that behavior change must be accepted and reinforced within a broad cultural context.

Guldan (1996) discussed obstacles to the success of community health promotion programs. Most relate to the ways interventions have been implemented such as the failure to engage target groups in the intervention, the failure to sustain interest in the intervention over time, and an inability to demonstrate the relevance of the intervention to the participants as individuals.

Kok (1993) offered three explanations for the ineffectiveness of many health promotion activities. First, not all health promotion interventions are sufficiently planned. Second, much of the applied research that is supposed to support health promotion theory and practice, is theory-based and not problem-based. Third, we often underestimate diffusion and adoption barriers in the implementation of health promotion interventions. We need to develop interventions to promote adoption of health promotion programs by policy makers.

Interventions succeed or fail because of politics. Most interventions originate through government or private foundation request for proposals (RFPs) that have allocated budgets to study and intervene to change some condition or set of behaviors, usually because it generates high financial costs and other inefficiencies. The RFPs are recruited by the funding agencies, and the grantees must follow guidelines outlined by the funding agencies. The nature and extent of the proposed interventions are limited by timelines and available funds. While an evaluation of the impact and cost effectiveness of an intervention is usually required by the funder, there is unspoken pressure to generate positive results, especially if the grantee wishes to receive funds for future projects. An intervention team creates a reputation for itself among funders for its creativity and effectiveness in creating significant behavior change. Politics and funding concerns, implicitly, if not explicitly, are part of every intervention plan and outcome (Fish and Leviton 1999; Gilliland and Taylor 1999); therefore, the structure and process of planning, funding, and implementing intervention projects tends to be paternalistic and protectionistic.

4.6 Discussion

There are at least three major constituents in every intervention, the intervener, the participant, and the fiscal sponsor. Other constituents, such as the participant's family, can also be involved depending on the nature of the intervention. Interveners are eager to establish a reputation for effecting statistically significant change. Funding sources are interested in furthering their goals and priorities and demonstrating to the public that they are testing innovative ideas toward solving pressing problems. Participants in interventions are a self-selected group with a mixture of personal, altruistic, and, in the case of paid volunteers, fiscal reasons for their involvement. All of these constituents have an eye on the outcome of the intervention. Indeed, some investigators stress that interventions should be as "potent" as possible to obtain measurable effects. Baranowski et al. (1997) suggested that we need to focus more on understanding underlying mechanisms and demonstrating how these mechanisms can affect outcome. Without a greater understanding of mediating or bridging variables, intervention outcomes will be short lived, in turn, causing interveners to look to imperfections in outcome methodology as the major problem.

According to Guldan (1996), and Last and Woolf (1996), there is a bias that successes, especially in health promotion, have been limited to individuals and groups who are more involved, well-educated, and middle class members of society. Those who respond poorly to health promotion interventions are the uneducated working class, the unemployed, the homeless, recent immigrants, and the disenfranchised. Because all of these groups suffer from poor health, even before health promotion is considered, health promotion tends to aggravate existing inequalities in health. Intervention successes, therefore, often are not generalizable to the general population (Glasgow et al. 1999).

4.7 Summary

Intervention, as previously noted, is an intrusion into value systems and is based on a relationship of mutual trust and shared expectations between the intervener and the participant. Too often, ethical considerations of an intervention focus on informed consent and the protection of interests. Researchers and clinicians must be aware that what transpires in the first meeting of the intervener and participant sets the stage for a successful or unsuccessful intervention. That first meeting is a mediating variable in the process of an intervention; it provides the opportunity to discuss mutual expectations regarding the intervention. Interveners tend to be paternalistic because they must follow a structured protocol to minimize bias. The degree of autonomy that the participant will have in the intervention should be discussed. Autonomy will vary with the nature of the intervention, but whatever the degree of autonomy, an intervention can succeed only if there is respect, openness, and trust between the intervener and the participant.

References

Baranowski, T. (1997). Families and health actions. In D. S. Gochman (Ed.), *Handbook of Health Behavior Research* (Vol. 1). New York: Plenum Press.

Baranowski, T., & Hearn, M. D. (1997). Health behavior interventions with families. In D. S. Gochman (Ed.), *Handbook of Health Behavior Research* (Vol. IV). New York: Plenum Press.

Baranowski, T., Lin, L. S., Wetter, D. W., Resnicow, K., & Hearn, M. D. (1997). Theory as mediating variables: Why aren't community interventions working as desired? *Annals of Epidemiology, 7*(S7), 589–595.

Baranowski, T., & Nader, P. R. (1985). Family involvement in health behavior change programs. In D. C. Turk & R. D. Kerns (Eds.), *Health, Illness, and Families: A Life-span Perspective.* New York: John Wiley.

Beach, M. C., Price, E. G., Gary, T. L., et al. (2005). Cultural competence: A systematic review of health care provider educational interventions. *Medical Care, 43*(4), 356–373.

Brach, C., & Fraser, I. (2000). Can cultural competency reduce social and ethnic health disparities? A review and conceptual model. *Med. Care Res. Rev, 57*(Suppl 1), 181–217.

Brown, F. H. (1991). The client as weaver. In F. H. Brown (Ed.), *Reweaving the Family Tapestry.* New York: W. W. Norton.

Bruhn, J. G. (1994). Social and psychological aspects of AIDS. In R. D. Muma, B. A. Lyons, J. M. Borucki, & R. B. Pollard (Eds.), *HIV Manual for Health Care Professionals.* Norwalk, CT: Appleton & Lange.

Bruhn, J. G., & Rebach, H. M. (1996). *Clinical Sociology: An Agenda for Action.* New York: Plenum Press.

Castro, F. G., Barrera, M, Jr, & Martinez, C. R, Jr. (2004). The cultural adaptation of preventive interventions: Resolving tension between fidelity and fit. *Preventive Science, 5*(1), 41–45.

Di Matteo, M. R. (1997). Health behaviors and care decisions: An overview of professional-patient communication. In D. S. Gochman (Ed.), *Handbook of Health Behavior Research* (Vol. II). New York: Plenum Press.

Fish, L., & Leviton, L. (1999). Program evaluation. In J. M. Raczynski & R. J. Di Clemente (Eds.), *Handbook of Health Promotion and Disease Prevention.* New York: Kluwer Academic/Plenum Publishers.

Fisher, T. L., Burnet, D. L., Huang, E. S., Chin, M. H., & Cagney, K. A. (2007). Cultural leverage: Interventions using culture to narrow racial disparities in health care. *Medical Care Research and Review, 64*(5 Suppl), 2435–2825.

Foeyt, J. P., Goodrick, G. K., & Gott, A. M. (1981). Limitation of behavioral treatment of obesity: Review and analysis. *Behavioral Medicine, 4,* 159–174.

Fraser, R. A. (1989). Social decision-making and the use of value management. *Ekistics, 56,* 171–174.

Gilliland, M. J., & Taylor, J. E. (1999). Planning community health interventions. In J. M. Raczynski & R. J. Di Clemente (Eds.), *Handbook of Health Promotion and Disease Prevention.* New York: Kluwer Academic/Plenum Publishers.

Glasgow, R. E., Vogt, T. M., & Boles, S. M. (1999). Evaluating the public health impact of health promotions interventions: The RE-AIM framework. *American Journal of Public Health, 89,* 1322–1327.

Gochman, D. S. (1997). Provider determinants of health behavior: An integration. In D. S. Gochman (Ed.), *Handbook of Health Behavior Research* (Vol. II). New York: Plenum Press.

Gorin, S. S., Badr, H., Krebs, P., & Das, P. (2012). Multilevel interventions and racial/ethnic health disparities. *Journal of National Cancer Institute Monographs, 2012*(44), 100–111.

Guldan, G. S. (1996). Obstacles to community health promotion. *Social Science and Medicine, 43,* 121–130.

Heller, K., Price, R. H., & Hogg, J. R. (1990). The role of social support in community and clinical interventions. In B. R. Sarason, I. G. Sarason, & G. R. Pierce (Eds.), *Social Support: An Interactional View.* New York: John Wiley.

Holmes, J. H., Lehman, A., Hade, E., et al. (2008). Challenges for multilevel health disparities research in a transdisciplinary environment. *American Journal of Preventive Medicine, 35*(2), S182–S192.

Jenkins, C. D. (1992). Assessment of outcomes of health intervention. *Social Science and Medicine, 35,* 367–375.

Kass, N. E. (2001). An ethics framework for public health. *American Journal of Public Health, 91*(11), 1776–1782.

Kline, M. V. (1999). Planning health promotion and disease prevention programs in multicultural populations. In R. M. Huff & M. V. Kline (Eds.), *Promoting Health in Multicultural Populations: A Handbook for Practitioners.* Thousand Oaks, CA: Sage.

Kok, G. (1993). Why are so many health promotion programs ineffective? *Health Promotion J Aust., 3*(2), 12–17.

Last, J., & Woolf, S. H. (1996). Ethical issues in health promotion and disease prevention. In S. H. Woolf, S. Jonas, & R. S. Lawrence (Eds.), *Health Promotion and Disease Prevention in Clinical Practice*. Baltimore: Williams and Wilkins.

Loewy, E. H. (1989). *Textbook of Medical Ethics*. New York: Plenum Press.

Masur, F. T. (1981). Adherence to health care regimens. In C. K. Prokop & L. A. Bradley (Eds.), *Medical Psychology: Contributions to Behavioral Medicine*. New York: Academic Press.

Oldenburg, B. F., Sallis, J. F., French, M. L., & Owen, N. (1999). Health promotion research and the diffusion and institutionalization of interventions. *Health Education Research, 14*, 121–130.

Oliver, T. R. (2006). The politics of public health policy. *Annual Review of Public Health, 27*, 195–233.

Paul, B. D. (Ed.). (1955). *Health, Culture, and Community: Case Studies of Public Reactions to Health Programs*. New York: Russell Sage Foundation.

Rolf, J. E., & Johnson, J. L. (1999). Opening doors to resilience intervention for prevention research. In M. D. Glantz & J. L. Johnson (Eds.), *Resilience and Development: Positive Life Adaptations*. New York: Plenum Publishers.

Rolland, J. S. (1994). *Families, Illness, and Disability: An Integrative Treatment Model*. New York: Basic Books.

Rosenthal, R., & Rosnow, R. L. (1975). *The Volunteer Subject*. New York: John Wiley.

Schalock, R. L. (1995). *Outcome-based Evaluation*. New York: Plenum Press.

Woodward, A., & Kawachi, I. (2000). Why reduce disparities? *Journal of Epidemiology and Community Health, 54*, 923–929.

Index

J. G. Bruhn, *Culture and Health Disparities*, SpringerBriefs in Public Health,
DOI: 10.1007/978-3-319-06462-8, © The Author(s) 2014